Advanced Practice in Nursing
Under the Auspices of the *International Council of Nurses (ICN)*

Series Editor
Christophe Debout
Chaire Santé Sciences-Po/IDS UMR Inserm 1145
Paris, France

This series of concise monographs, endorsed by the International Council of Nurses, explores various aspects of advanced nursing practice at the international level.

The ICN International Nurse Practitioner/Advanced Practice Nursing Network definition has been adopted for this series to define advanced nursing practice: "A Nurse Practitioner/Advanced Practice Nurse is a registered nurse who has acquired the expert knowledge base, complex decision-making skills and clinical competencies for expanded practice, the characteristics of which are shaped by the context and/or country in which s/he is credentialed to practice. A master's degree is recommended for entry level."

At the international level, advanced nursing practice encompasses two professional profiles:

Nurse practitioners (NPs) who have mastered advanced nursing practice, and are capable of diagnosing, making prescriptions for and referring patients. Though they mainly work in the community, some also work in hospitals.

Clinical nurse specialists (CNSs) are expert nurses who deliver high-quality nursing care to patients and promote quality care and performance in nursing teams.

The duties performed by these two categories of advanced practice nurses on an everyday basis can be divided into five interrelated roles:

Clinical practice
Consultation
Education
Leadership
Research

The series addresses four topics directly related to advanced nursing practice:
APN in practice (NPs and CNSs)
Education and continuous professional development for advanced practice nurses
Managerial issues related to advanced nursing practice
Policy and regulation of advanced nursing practice

The contributing authors are mainly APNs (NPs and CNSs) recruited from the ICN International Nurse Practitioner/Advanced Practice Nursing Network. They include clinicians, educators, researchers, regulators and managers, and are recognized as experts in their respective fields.

Each book within the series reflects the fundamentals of nursing/advanced nursing practice and will promote evidence-based nursing.

More information about this series at http://www.springer.com/series/13871

Madrean Schober

Introduction to Advanced Nursing Practice

An International Focus

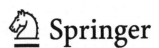

Madrean Schober
Schober Global Healthcare Consulting
Indianapolis
Indiana
USA

Advanced Practice in Nursing
ISBN 978-3-319-32203-2   ISBN 978-3-319-32204-9   (eBook)
DOI 10.1007/978-3-319-32204-9

Library of Congress Control Number: 2016955805

Printed on acid-free paper

This Springer imprint is published by Springer Nature
The registered company is Springer International Publishing AG Switzerland

Foreword

Advanced nursing practice can mean many things to many people. These highly knowledgeable and skilled nurses are increasing in popularity as a solution to many of the challenges that healthcare faces today: advances in technology, the increasing complexity of health services, structural changes in healthcare delivery, and changing healthcare needs. The need for a more flexible and cost-effective approach to the delivery of care has never been more appropriate, as the needs of disadvantaged communities and vulnerable populations are being addressed.

In order to understand this role and its importance throughout the globe, it is necessary to examine and compare the role in a variety of international contexts. In Introduction to Advanced Nursing Practice: An International Focus, Madrean Schober takes a wide-angle snapshot of the landscape of advanced nursing practice (ANP) across the globe. Starting with the origins of the role, this book highlights the drivers which led to the development of ANP in various countries and how the position has been influenced by international organizations, such as the International Council of Nurses.

With case studies from every continent, Introduction to Advanced Nursing Practice discusses some of the controversial issues such as prescribing, diagnoses, and hospital privileges. It takes a hard look at competencies and task reallocation and addresses the development of education for this role, including teaching methods and clinical practice. Regulation, accreditation, certification, and licensure, are also examined, along with frameworks and models of professional regulation from the USA, New Zealand, Scotland, and Ireland.

Advanced practice nurses are skilled in assessing individuals, families, and community health needs and diagnosing the need for nursing intervention. Their preparation allows them to provide integrated care, including disease management, making or receiving referrals, or supervising and guiding other caregivers. How the APN role interconnects within healthcare systems and between other healthcare professionals is an important part of this book, which also looks at the challenges of professional conflict and public acceptance of the role.

Advanced practice nurses are capable of planning and implementing programs to promote the health of communities, and they are prepared in the methodology of research that enables a critical look at the quality, relevance and outcomes of care, and can use this to improve practice and expand services. This role can open up many career paths, and this publication looks at the professional progression up the clinical career ladder, including scopes of practice, performance reviews, and evaluation.

Covering all aspects of this role, this book also looks at the importance of research and how we can strengthen the advanced nursing practice agenda. It is high time for a thorough examination of this role across the globe, and this is exactly what this impressive book provides. I am delighted that such a thought-provoking, analytical review of advanced nursing practice has finally been published.

Geneva, Switzerland   Dr Judith Shamian
                                          President of the International Council of Nurses

Preface

The launching of the International Council of Nurses' International Nurse Practitioner/Advanced Practice Nursing Network in 2000 signaled the beginning of a new era in the recognition of the progression of advanced nursing practice worldwide. Long thought to be the realm of professional practice in the United States, it seemed development of advanced practice nursing roles was on its way to travel around the globe. Representatives from 25 countries, displaying their national flags, gathered for the Network launching to provide encouragement, inspiration, and energy for what had become an international phenomenon. Since that time, enthusiasm for advanced nursing practice continues and interest in the advancement of nursing has progressed.

Increased visibility revealed uncertainty as to the intent and function of this new category of nurses. The International Council of Nurses observed this situation and took the first step in 2002 to recommend a definition, scope of practice, and characteristics for a nurse practicing in an advanced capacity and role. The intent was to present an international benchmark to refer to and thus encourage countries to discuss and develop the concept sensitive to their national context. Since that time the discipline of advanced nursing practice has grown, discussions have become more highly developed, and research on the subject has increased.

Built on the growing body of knowledge and maturing nature of advanced nursing, this book is intended to be a resource for healthcare professionals and key decision makers. Chapter 1 provides an overview of advanced nursing practice. The overview includes a definition, characteristics, and assumptions associated with advanced practice. The growing presence of advanced nursing practice is acknowledged in Chap. 2. In addition to identifying the impetus behind national initiatives, this chapter provides in-depth profiles of country-specific development. Chapter 3 describes the nature of advanced practice nursing including the significance of reaching consensus on a designated and context appropriate title. Principles of education for these advanced nursing roles are presented in Chap. 4. Dimensions of role and practice development comprise Chap. 5 followed by the essence of professional regulation in Chap. 6. Challenges when introducing this category of nurse into the healthcare workforce and strategies to face issues that might be brought into question are discussed in Chap. 7. Professional progression and career pathways that integrate advanced practice nurses into the healthcare workforce are suggested in Chap. 8. Chapter 9 depicts the essential nature and significance of research that promotes and supports advanced nursing practice. Finally, the concluding chapter proposes consideration of an agenda for the future.

The author draws on extensive personal international experience with country initiatives and close association with the continually evolving ICN International Nurse Practitioner/Advanced Practice Nursing Network. In addition, selectively chosen key country and regional representatives, literature and unpublished sources complement the experiences of the author. Key informants have been chosen on the basis that they are formal or informal leaders, persons in positions of authority or experts who have knowledge of role development in their respective countries or regions. For some this is the first time they have portrayed advanced nursing practice development in their country. The enthusiasm and passion of the author for this topic has contributed to the writing of this publication along with a sense of amazement in observing the international evolution of nursing that has taken place in the past 15–20 years.

I am thankful to a number of people who in various ways have contributed to the resonant and extensive nature of this volume on Advanced Nursing Practice. Most importantly, I want to express my sincere gratitude to country and regional representatives who willingly shared stories of role development and in many cases translated the narrative from their first language to English for this publication. This has provided greater depth and understanding of the expansive and worldwide nature of advanced nursing development. I am also indebted to Fadwa Affara, who willingly and generously gave of her time and expertise to review content and provide comment for each chapter. Not only was Fadwa the lead International Council of Nurses' consultant for the launching of the ICN International Nurse Practitioner/ Advanced Practice Nursing Network in 2000 but she also continues to campaign tirelessly at an international level for the professional advancement of nursing.

Indianapolis, IN, USA   Madrean Schober, PhD, MSN, ANP, FAANP

Contents

Overview of Advanced Nursing Practice

Abstract

The field of advanced nursing practice and diverse levels of advanced nursing is a growing trend worldwide in the provision of a variety of healthcare services. This chapter introduces the concept of advanced nursing practice by offering an international definition and key characteristics of an advanced practice nurse. Assumptions that should be found wherever nursing exists are identified as the foundation for progressing to advanced levels of nursing. Topics to consider when forging a new nursing role are discussed along with country issues that shape advanced nursing practice development.

Keywords

Advanced nursing practice • Advanced practice nurse • Definition • Characteristics • Country issues • Assumptions

The field of advanced nursing practice (ANP) and diverse levels of advanced nursing is a growing trend worldwide in the provision of a variety of healthcare services. This chapter introduces the concept of ANP by offering an international definition and key characteristics of an advanced practice nurse (APN). Assumptions that should be found wherever nursing exists are identified as the foundation for progressing to advanced levels of nursing practice. In addition, topics to consider when forging a new nursing role are discussed along with country issues that shape ANP development.

The terms "advanced nursing practice" and "advanced practice nursing" are often used interchangeably in reference to advanced nursing roles or advanced levels of nursing practice. Lacking an international consensus on the use of terminology, the terms "advanced nursing practice" (ANP) for the purpose of this publication will refer comprehensively to the discipline or this entire field of nursing and "advanced practice nursing" (APN) and "advanced practice nurse" (APN) will refer

© Springer International Publishing Switzerland 2016
M. Schober, *Introduction to Advanced Nursing Practice*,
DOI 10.1007/978-3-319-32204-9_1

to a specific role, the nurse that practices in that role, specific education, and specific professional regulation relevant to the nurse. These definitions are consistent with language used by the Canadian Nurses Association [1] national framework for ANP and the Scottish ANP Toolkit [11] that has provided guidance [12] to the other countries in the United Kingdom (England, Northern Ireland, and Wales) and in an earlier publication [10] written under the auspices of ICN. The comprehensive use of ANP, as an umbrella term, includes but is not limited in reference to country-specific titles such as nurse practitioner, clinical nurse specialist, and advanced practice nurse practitioner. Chapter 3, Nature of Practice, provides a more in-depth discussion of the use of designated titles for APN roles. The following section offers an international definition and profile for an APN.

1.1   Definition and Profile of an Advanced Practice Nurse

During the 1990s, the International Council of Nurses (ICN) observed the growing presence of ANP as countries reviewed their healthcare systems and looked for new alternatives for the provision of healthcare services. In an effort to keep up with increasing demands and economic limitations, it appeared that there was better acceptance of new nursing roles and practice models [10]. Since the time ICN began noting the presence of APN roles, there has been an increasing consensus that APNs are effective and beneficial when integrated into a variety of healthcare systems [2, 5, 14].

Noting a need to improve visibility and international representation of the emerging ANP discipline, ICN launched the International Nurse Practitioner/Advanced Practice Nursing Network (INP/APNN) in 2000. This event followed collaboration of representatives from the United Kingdom and the United States who had already initiated conferences in 1993 to begin to embody a global identity for ANP. The governing structure of a Core Steering Group and seven subgroups was established for the Network along with a web site (http://www.icn-apnetwork.org). As the Network has evolved, international representation has increased, ANP-focused conferences take place every two years, and ongoing research in the field of ANP is promoted. A more in-depth description of INP/APNN can be found on the Network web site and in Chap. 2.

Simultaneously as the Network was established and in the process of international dialogue, confusion rather than consensus emerged when trying to define and characterize the APN role. In an attempt to explain the nature of this nursing role, ICN took the first step by providing a definition in 2002 [6]. A recommendation for scope of practice and suggestions to guide development of standards for professional regulation, education, and competencies subsequently followed [7]. The ICN publication serves as a benchmark for international discussion on the concept of ANP and APN roles. Significant development has occurred in the field since the launching of INP/APNN and the release of this landmark document. However, literature continues to confirm not only growth in the presence of APNs but also a continued theme of uncertainty in defining ANP [3, 4, 8, 9]. This publication, written under the auspices of ICN, continues to facilitate the discourse on a dynamic and growing nursing discipline.

1.1.1 Definition

Clear definitions are essential to identifying and positioning a profession within a healthcare system [13]. In offering a definition for the APN role, ICN acknowledged that country milieu shapes role development and provided the following definition as a point of reference for discussion:

> [The] APN is a registered nurse who has acquired the expert knowledge base, complex decision-making skills and clinical competencies for expanded practice, the characteristics of which are shaped by the context and/or country in which s/he is credentialed to practice. A master's degree is recommended for entry level. (ICN [6] and [7] p. 29)

In order to provide a profile of the APN role, ICN offered also a delineation of APN characteristics. These characteristics follow in Sect. 1.1.2.

1.1.2 Characteristics of the Advanced Practice Nurse

In order to support and add to the APN definition, ICN identified characteristics of an APN and provided the following recommendations:

- Educational preparation
    - Educational preparation beyond generalist nursing education
    - Formal recognition of educational programs preparing for the advanced practice nursing role (accredited or approved)
    - Formal system of licensure, registration, certification, and credentialing
- Nature of Practice
    - The ability to Integrate research [evidence based practice], education and clinical management
    - High degree of professional autonomy and independent practice
    - Case management/[manage] own caseload at an advanced level
    - Advanced assessment, decision-making skills and diagnostic reasoning skills
    - Recognized advanced clinical competencies
    - The ability to provide consultant services to other healthcare professionals
    - Plans, implements and evaluates programs
    - Recognized first point of contact for clients
- Regulatory mechanisms – Country specific professional regulation underpins APN practice
    - Right to diagnose
    - Authority to prescribe medications and treatments
    - Authority to refer clients to other professionals
    - Authority to admit patients to hospital
    - Officially recognized titles for nurses working in advanced practice roles
    - Legislation to confer and protect the title (e.g. nurse practitioner, advanced practice nurse, clinical nurse specialist)
    - Legislation, policies or some form of regulatory mechanism specific to advanced practice nurses

(Adapted from ICN [7], p. 29)

The definition and characteristics offered by ICN are necessarily broad given the necessity to take into consideration variations in healthcare systems, regulatory mechanisms, and nursing education in individual countries. Since the release of the ICN publication in 2008, the ANP discipline has matured with the APN increasingly seen as a clinical expert with characteristics of the role crosscutting over numerous themes that include understanding of issues of governance, policy development, and clinical leadership. As a result, promoting leadership as an aspect of the APN role has become increasingly important. Integration of research knowledge and skills has also become more central to role education and development.

In spite of a lack of consensus in attempting to define APN roles, certain conditions supportive of ANP exist wherever nursing is present. These assumptions are identified next in Sect. 1.1.3.

1.1.3   Assumptions: The Foundation for Advanced Nursing Practice

There are key components for ANP that should be found wherever nursing exists and that provide the foundation for the development of advanced levels of nursing practice. The following assumptions provide points for international consideration and dialogue. All APNs:

- are practitioners of nursing providing safe and competent patient care
- have their foundation in registered generalist nurse education
- have roles which require formal education beyond the preparation of the generalist nurse
- have roles of increased levels of competency that are measurable
- have competencies which address the ethical, legal, care giving and professional development of the advanced practice role
- have competencies and standards which are periodically reviewed for maintaining currency in practice
- are influenced by the global, social, political, economic and technological milieu

(ICN [7] p. 11)

The position of ICN emphasizes that:

The degree of judgment, skill, knowledge and accountability increases between the preparation of nurse generalists and that of the APN. This added breadth and depth of practice is achieved through additional education and experience in clinical practice; however, the core does not change and it remains the context of nursing. (ICN [7] p. 9)

Further in-depth discussion of titles, role characteristics, scope of practice, and competencies can be found in Chap. 3: Nature of Practice. Section 1.2 highlights issues to consider when undertaking the ANP concept.

1.2   Forging a New Nursing Role

Forging a new nursing role when there are no role models in place highlights issues for debate and discussion. The following questions require consideration when exploring and progressing with the ANP concept:

- What is the nurses' perspective of advancement and advanced nursing practice?
- What does advancement or professional progression for nursing mean within the country?
- Is there a career structure for promotion that could support the integration of advanced practice nurses?
- Is there an official place for the APN within the healthcare system with well-defined job descriptions and a career pathway commensurate to their qualifications and capabilities?
- Are the key components of APN practice acknowledged and addressed?

1.2.1   Country Issues that Shape Development

The fundamental level of nursing practice and access to an adequate level of nursing education that exists in a country shapes the potential for introducing and developing the APN role. The professional status of nursing and its ability to introduce a new role will influence the launching of an ANP scheme. The prominence and maturity of nursing can be assessed by the presence of other nursing specialties, levels of nursing education, policies specific to nurses, and the extent of nursing research (F. Affara, 18 February 2016, personal communication).

Conclusion

International enthusiasm for advanced nursing practice has increased. The result is increased visibility of this concept and associated advanced practice nursing roles. However, there is a need to offer clarity, guidelines, and resources for key stakeholders, decision makers, healthcare planners, administrators, and professionals as they proceed to explore advanced practice nursing roles as an option for provision of healthcare services. This chapter offers a definition and role characteristics for the advanced practice nurse as a point of reference to facilitate discussion. Key issues to consider when coordinating, planning, or launching an advanced nursing practice initiative are suggested.

References

1. Canadian Nurses Association (CNA) (2008) Advanced nursing practice: a national framework. CNA, Ottawa
2. Delemaire M, LaFortune G (2010) Nurses in advanced roles: a description and evaluation of experiences in 12 developed countries. OECD Health Working Papers, No. 54, OECD Publishing. doi:10.1787/5kmbrcfms5g7-en

3. Donald F, Bryant-Lukosius D, Martin-Misener R, Kaasalainen S, Kilpatrick K, Carter N, Harbman P, Bourgeault I, DiCenso A (2010) Clinical nurse specialists and nurse practitioners: title confusion and lack of role clarity, Nurs Leadersh 23 (Special Issue) pp. 189–210
4. Gardner G, Chang A, Duffield C (2007) Making nursing work: breaking through the role confusion of advanced practice nursing. JAN 57(4):383–391
5. Horrocks S, Anderson E, Salisbury C (2002) Systematic review on whether nurse practitioners working in primary care can provide equivalent care to doctors. BMJ 324:819–823
6. International Council of Nurses (ICN) (2002) Definition and characteristics of the role. Retrieved 19 February 2016 from http://www.icn-apnetwork.org
7. International Council of Nurses (ICN) (2008) The scope of practice, standards and competencies of the advanced practice nurse, ICN Regulation Series. ICN, Geneva
8. Pulcini J, Jelic M, Gul R, Loke AY (2010) An international survey on advanced practice nursing education, practice and regulation. Journal of Nursing Scholarship 42(1):31–39
9. Sastre-Fullana P, De Pedro-Gomez JE, Bennasar-Veny M, Serrano-Gallardo P, Morales-Ascencio JM (2014) Competency frameworks for advanced practice nursing: a literature review. INR 61(4):534–542
10. Schober M, Affara F (2006) Advanced nursing practice. Blackwell Publishing Ltd, Oxford
11. Scottish Government (2008) Supporting the development of advanced nursing practice: a toolkit approach. Scottish Government, CNO Directorate
12. Scottish Government (2010) Advanced nursing practice roles: guidance for NHS boards. Scottish Government
13. Styles MM, Affara FA (1997) ICN on regulation: towards a 21st century model. International Council of Nurses, Geneva
14. Ter Maten-Speksnijder A, Grypdonck M, Pool A, Meurs P, van Staa AL (2013) A literature review of the Dutch debate on the nurse practitioner role: efficiency vs. professional development. INR 61:44–54

A Growing Presence

2

Abstract

The development of advanced nursing practice has caught international attention as healthcare planners and key decision makers explore options to meet the increasingly diverse healthcare needs of the world's populations. One solution for enhancing healthcare services in institutional settings and primary care is the inclusion of advanced practice nurses in the healthcare workforce. The integration of these relatively new nursing roles presents a dynamic change in thinking for healthcare professionals and the systems in which they practice. This chapter describes the growing presence of advanced nursing practice internationally, identifies drivers that motivate consideration of advanced nursing roles and provides wide-ranging and in-depth examples of country specific development. In addition, the extent and relevance of international support for advanced nursing practice is described.

Keywords

International support • Country profiles • Development patterns • Drivers • Motivation

The development of advanced nursing practice (ANP) has caught international attention as healthcare planners and key decision makers explore options to meet the increasingly diverse healthcare needs of the world's populations [19, 40, 43, 75, 116]. One solution for enhancing healthcare services in institutional settings and primary care is the inclusion of advanced practice nurses (APN) in the healthcare workforce. The integration of these relatively new nursing roles presents a dynamic change in thinking for healthcare professionals and the systems in which they practice. This chapter describes the growing presence of ANP internationally, identifies drivers that motivate consideration of advanced nursing roles, and provides wide-ranging examples of country specific development. In addition, the extent of international support for ANP and the various levels and types of APN roles that are emerging is described.

Advanced practice nurses obtain advanced knowledge and skills beyond their initial general/basic nursing registration. Through advanced education they are able to practice at an advanced clinical level in a wide range of settings such as specialty wards in hospitals, primary healthcare, specialized clinics, general practitioner surgeries, and rural and remote settings (see Chap. 1 for APN role definition and characteristics and Chap. 3 for an in-depth discussion on Nature of Practice). The International Council of Nurses (ICN) began to take note of the growing presence of ANP in the 1990s. Factors contributing to a greater demand for an expanding nursing scope of practice were presented at a conference in Adelaide, Australia, in 2002 organized by the ICN International Nurse Practitioner/Advanced Practice Nursing Network [118]. International surveys conducted from 2001 to 2014 found that anywhere from 25 to 60 countries were in various stages of exploring or implementing APN roles [64, 109, 112, 116].

2.1   Incentives and Motivation for Advanced Nursing Practice

Nurses in advanced practice roles are increasingly viewed as a vital part of the healthcare workforce. This section identifies and describes the motivation or incentive leading decision makers to investigate and pursue the concept of ANP and associated APN roles.

In a review of data based papers and policy reports, De Geest et al. [39] identified five drivers that influence APN role development:

- The healthcare needs of the population
- Education (for nurses)
- Workforce issues
- Practice patterns and new models of care
- Legal and policy context

Findings from this review suggest that the potential role for an APN is shaped by country context and thus deserves an assessment in advance of the specific setting and milieu in which an APN will practice. In a study reviewing the development of APNs in 12 countries, Delamaire and LaFortune [40] provided the following main factors motivating introduction of APN roles in a select group of countries:

- Promote higher quality care
- Contain cost of care
- Enhance career prospects in the nursing profession

In a comprehensive literature review conducted by Schober [121] to assess the momentum behind ANP initiatives, four main themes were identified:

- An identified healthcare need for service provision
- An answer to skill mix and healthcare workforce planning
- A desire for the advancement of nursing roles to enhance professional development
- Public demand for improved access to healthcare delivery

Similar to findings by De Geest et al. [39] and Delamaire and LaFortune [40], Schober [121] found that an identified population need for healthcare services, workforce planning, and practice patterns, and/or a desire for new models of healthcare provision emerged as significant incentives for consideration of APN roles. What is of particular interest is a view that APN roles are associated with a path for professional and career advancement. This perspective was seen as a way to increase the attractiveness of the nursing profession and retain expert nurses in clinical practice [40, 121]. In a study conducted in Singapore, enhancing the status of nursing was identified as the primary driver initially for promoting ANP [121].

2.2   Patterns and Drivers of Advanced Nursing Practice Development

Advanced nursing practice schemes for introducing and integrating APNs into the healthcare workforce are context sensitive to the situational realities in which the concept emerges. The culture of healthcare service delivery, sociopolitical environment, and the awareness of ANP by key influential stakeholders and decision makers provide a composite background for the consideration, introduction, and development of APN roles.

2.2.1   Launching an Advanced Nursing Practice Initiative

No single starting point is seen as pivotal when investigating the value of ANP and its place in a country's healthcare workforce. Section 2.1 identifies drivers that have stimulated interest in APN roles, but motivation alone does not speak to the complexities and numerous factors that require consideration in launching a successful ANP scheme. Issues associated with the nursing culture, educational options for nurses, regulatory/policy infrastructure, financial/human resources, and systems of healthcare delivery ultimately must come together to lend support to the accompanying changes that are required. Based on the literature [39, 40, 116, 121, 122, 127] experiences of the author and country profiles provided in this publication, the following factors appear to provide a strong foundation for launching a successful ANP initiative:

- An identified need for APN roles, frequently based on population needs for healthcare services.
- Strong education programs for the generalist/basic nurse that provide a robust foundation for a nurse to pursue advanced education.
- Flexible and pragmatic education alternatives that not only educate competent APNs but offer options to bridge the gaps in nursing education when a country is in a transitional stage in program development, e.g., when basic nursing education leading to preparation at an advanced level is lacking, courses/modules are made available to fill the gaps in education.
- Clinical career pathways or clinical ladders for professional progression.
- Available APN role models and effective mentorship. In the absence of role models, observation of role models in countries with APN success or recruiting APNs on a short term basis can be an interim consideration.
- Presence of effective influential nursing leadership at the governmental, ministry of health, regulatory agency, health department levels.
- Access to international consultant expertise that is continuous and sustainable.
- The ability of agencies and organizations to work together when coordinating integration of APNs in the healthcare workforce.

This list is not suggested as a recipe for success but an identification of factors to consider. One country's success or limitations are not necessarily transferable to another country but can provide exemplars of essential features to take into account. In this chapter, Sects. 2.2.2, 2.2.3, 2.2.4, and 2.2.5 describe country profiles associated with an identified driver that motivated country interest in ANP. Additional country profiles are presented in Sect. 2.4 and offer the reader a comprehensive and in-depth understanding of the variance in country based schemes. It is worth noting that a country profile of ANP development may vary by state or province or within individual institutions within the same country. This approach occurs when choices are made to adopt policies that are specific to circumstances, healthcare settings, and delivery systems. In addition, a country profile can vary somewhat depending on the national representative providing the description.

2.2.2   Nursing Education as the Origin

The term advanced nursing brings to mind the call for additional or a higher level of education to prepare the APN. As mentioned earlier in the chapter, the motivation to establish advanced nursing education was identified as a common starting point for an ANP initiative. Sections 2.2.2.1 and 2.2.2.2 provide two examples of that approach. The country profiles also demonstrate how the future for ANP is intrinsically linked to the nursing culture and level of nursing education available and accessible in the country.

2.2.2.1 Pakistan: Advancing Nursing Education

As part of the nursing development at Aga Khan University (AKU) in Karachi, Pakistan, a 2-year Master of Science in Nursing (MScN) was established in 2001 with five students. National and international experts developed the foundation for a curriculum based on "The Essentials of Master's Education for Advanced Practice Nursing" [3]. The aim was to prepare nurse leaders in education, evidence based clinical practice, and administration. The program took a generalist approach with emphasis on research and advanced clinical practice. In 2008, in addition to inclusion of clinical experience, education and administration practicums were introduced.

Based on the Pakistani adaptation of the AACN [3] model, the MScN curriculum was conceptualized on three major components: (1) graduate nursing core content with content suitable for all students, (2) advanced practice nurse content for students who will provide clinical services, and (3) cognate courses with content linked to student interest in their potential practice. The program was offered as full time or part time with opportunities for multidisciplinary learning via elective courses from other AKU graduate programs. Students were provided with funding for research in support of their MScN thesis.

However, the picture for evolution of nursing and ANP in Pakistan has been uneven. Since the founding of Pakistan in 1947, nursing development has been challenging albeit strengthened under substandard conditions. In order to understand the status of ANP, a brief history of the establishment of nursing provides the country context. The first nursing school, established in Pakistan in 1948, offered a 3-year general nursing program, but by 1952 only seven nurses were qualified from this program. The school was spearheaded by a physician, the medical superintendent of the hospital with which the school was affiliated. The first post-basic education programs to prepare nurses for teaching and ward administration were started in 1956. Over the next three decades, one college remained the single source of nursing education at the post-basic level [60], even though the demand for more nurse teachers and managers was growing due to a steady increase in the number of hospitals and nursing schools offering basic education. In the 1980s, the number of nursing colleges grew from one to five but was limited to the public sector of the country.

The first post-RN BScN and the first 4-year BScN were implemented in 1988 and 1997, respectively, at the Aga Khan University (AKU). Subsequently, in 2001 the first Master of Science in Nursing (MScN) program was established at AKU. Also, at this time, one of the nursing colleges in the public sector affiliated with a provincial university began to offer a post-RN BScN degree. In the next 15 years, rapid growth occurred in the number of nursing schools and colleges offering undergraduate nursing degree programs in the country. However, until 2010, the Aga Khan University remained the only institution in the country to prepare graduate level nurses due to the lack of PhD prepared nurse educators.

At Aga Khan University, the curriculum of the MScN program was grounded in the advanced practice framework with courses to prepare nurses as leaders in nursing practice with advanced knowledge and skills for their roles in either urban, rural, tertiary-care, or community settings. However, considering the potential pool of candidates for this program, additional courses were added to enhance the teaching and leadership competencies of the graduates. Because of the limited pool of BScN prepared nurses at that time and very limited funding opportunities for higher education for nurses, the program consisted of five or fewer students in each cohort until 2005. Gradually, with the increase of BScN graduates from the 4-year BScN, the intake of MScN increased. For the initial several years, most of the graduates took an educator role after completion of the MScN due to a high demand for graduate level prepared nurses in nursing schools and colleges. As of 2015, 116 students have graduated with 66% working as educators and 25% in clinical administration.

Pakistan is one of the very few countries in the world that has an inverse ratio of registered nurses (90,276) to registered physicians (175,223) [102]. Although nurses and midwives play a significant role worldwide in the delivery of healthcare services, their potential has not yet been fully realized in Pakistan. Higher education has remained mostly inaccessible to the majority of nurses in the country [146]. (R. Gul, Acting Dean, School of Nursing and Midwifery, Aga Khan University, Pakistan, 06 April 2016, personal communication)

2.2.2.2 ANP Development in Switzerland: Visions and Reality

Advanced nursing practice (ANP) education was introduced in Switzerland in the year 2000 with the first Master of Science in Nursing program at the Institute of Nursing Science at the University of Basel [68]. The gradual replacement of non-Master prepared nurses in clinical specialist roles (Höfa 1 &2) [133] and the development of other Master of Nursing Science curricula at various institutes of higher education starting from 2004 further stimulated the implementation of ANP roles in various clinical settings in Switzerland. In 2012, a definition of ANP based on the ICN definition [117, 136] was released. Initial research to evaluate ANP roles and models has been undertaken [66, 72, 91, 95, 126, 144] and a framework for ANP practice evaluation has been published [16]. At the policy level the ANP roles are not yet legally protected and formally accredited; however, legislation to regulate healthcare professions such as nursing, physiotherapy, midwifery, and occupational therapy at the bachelor's and master's level throughout Switzerland is in progress [55].

Definition of APN in Switzerland

The Swiss Nursing Association, in collaboration with the Swiss Association for Nursing Science (ANF), SwissANP, and the University Institute for Nursing Education and Research in Lausanne developed a definition of an advanced practice nurse (APN) in 2012 to provide clarity among all stakeholders on ANP [117, 136] using the International Council of Nurses definition as a basis [122]. Working as an APN in Switzerland requires a minimum level of master's education by this definition [39, 117].

Education for ANP

The first Master of Science in Nursing study program pursuing ANP was launched in Switzerland at the Institute of Nursing Science, Faculty of Medicine, University of Basel in 2000. The study program and its curriculum were developed on the basis of internationally recognized ANP competencies [57] and has inspired subsequent similar programs in Switzerland (UNIL 2006; universities of applied sciences of Bern, St. Gallen, and Zurich, including the private Kalaidos University of Applied Sciences beginning in 2004) [11, 52, 67, 69, 71, 150] and the German speaking countries in the past few years. As of May 2016, 274 nurses graduated within one of the Swiss Master in Nursing Science programs (German speaking based programs). As a result of feedback from INS master's alumni who highlighted the need for further advanced level clinical education, the postgraduate program *Diploma of Advanced Studies ANP-plus* (ANPplus) was developed. This program, which started in 2012 at INS (INS ANPplus), prepares nurses for an NP role and paved the way for the expansion to this specific ANP role in the Swiss setting.

Swiss ANP Research

Although evaluation studies of ANP roles or models of care with APN involvement in Switzerland exist [14, 66, 72, 90, 91, 95, 110, 111, 126, 144, 151–153], investment in ANP outcome evaluation is key for the future. Recently, an ANP evaluation framework was developed and published to guide these efforts [18]. Published outcome evaluations so far focus on elderly patients with multiple illnesses in hospital or ambulatory hospital care, HIV care, and primary care, and confirm the positive outcomes of advanced nursing practice reported internationally on process and outcome parameters. A study evaluating ANP in lung cancer care is in progress [126]. More specifically, a recent study in an urban walk-in clinic revealed that more than 50 % of specific patient care needs could be covered within the advanced nursing scope of practice; the authors concluded that "assigning APNs to primary care clinics would contribute a meaningful new professional role to Switzerland's healthcare system" [72]. In terms of outcome research, the evaluation of comprehensive services offered by ANP teams showed shorter length of hospitalization for patients, increased self-efficacy, and work satisfaction for nurses in the acute geriatric setting [144] and increased adherence to medications in the ambulatory setting [95]. In a qualitative study, patients stated that in an APN-led program, they were taken seriously and learned how to cope with consequences of multiple chronic diseases [91]. An in-home health consultation program by APNs resulted in less acute medical events, falls and fall related injuries and hospitalizations [66]. However, economic analyses are currently missing in the Swiss setting.

Swiss Policy on APN

At the policy level, the interest in APN roles has grown, especially in light of the shortage of primary care physicians and the development of new care models [8, 54, 77]. There is an interest within the nursing profession to develop a legal framework for ANP. Despite this growing interest within and outside the nursing profession, initiatives for legally defining APN or accrediting APN have so far not been successful. Legislation to regulate healthcare professions at the tertiary level throughout Switzerland is in progress [55, 137, 138]. While the regulation of competencies on the bachelor's level was not questioned, including the master's level into the law was disputed and future discussions are necessary.

Summary and Prospects

While being late in ANP development compared to some other Anglo-Saxon countries, Switzerland, and especially the Institute of Nursing Science at the University of Basel, has taken a leading position in the German-speaking world in view of ANP education and role development since 2000. Starting with a master's program for Nursing Science at University level as a main driver for ANP development in 2000, the new role has been taken up swiftly by many hospitals, nursing homes, and recently also primary care settings. ANP evaluation research is underway. Despite increasing numbers of APNs operating in the Swiss healthcare setting, legislation lags behind and legal provisions to regulate master's programs in nursing as well as APN professional practice are still to be established. (K. Fierz, R. Schwendimann, M. Henry, O. Mauthner, H. Stoll, D. Nicca, S. De Geest, Institute of Nursing Science, University of Basel, Basel, Switzerland, 18 May 2016, personal communication)

The author notes that development described in this profile pertains mainly to the German speaking part of Switzerland and acknowledges that there is early development in Lausanne, the French speaking part of the country, for a specialist nursing clinical practitioner. The University of Lausanne (UNIL) http://www.unil.ch/index.html and the University of Applied Sciences Western Switzerland (HES-SO) http://www.hes-so.ch/ are offering a joint Master of Science in Nursing Sciences. At the time of writing the author did not have an in-depth profile describing this program.

2.2.3   Shortage of Healthcare Professionals

A response to identified population healthcare needs accentuated by projected shortages of healthcare professionals, specifically physicians, was found to be a common reason for the introduction of APNs [39, 40, 121]. Fragmented healthcare delivery and limited access to healthcare services were commonly associated with a shortage of healthcare professionals, particularly physicians. Providing an historical background and timeframe to benchmark against, the trajectory of United States development begins this section but is not identified as a country profile. The demand for highly skilled nurses in hospital settings and a physician shortage in the United States led to the introduction of the APN (now called advanced practice registered nurse [APRN]) roles in the country. As nurses embraced expertise from medicine and other disciplines, the expanded nursing roles became more visible and developed under four categories: certified registered nurse anesthetists (CRNA), certified nurse midwives (CNMW), clinical nurse specialists (CNS), and nurse practitioners (NP) [74, 134]. An increasing number of NPs and their success in providing primary care services since the 1960s rapidly escalated success. As of November 2015, the American Association of Nurse Practitioners indicated that there were more than 205,000 licensed NPs in the United States [5]. Even though there are four categories of APRNs in the country, it is the increased visibility of the NP role that provides an historical benchmark for other countries wanting to emulate this success. Similarly, the following profiles describe responses to an anticipated shortage of physicians and/or identified heavy workload for general practitioners.

2.2.3.1 Nurse Practitioners in the Netherlands: Response to a Physician Shortage

The Netherlands has nearly 20 years of experience in developing the Dutch experience of the nurse practitioner (NP) (Dutch title is "nurse specialist"). The following example provides a timeline of progress, data on NPs in the country and a description of the evolvement of ANP.

The NP was introduced in the Netherlands in 1997. The main reason to start this task reallocation within the Dutch healthcare system was a projected shortage of physicians. Since their introduction until 2016, NPs are trained in a dual education system, i.e., an educational program that combines apprenticeships in a healthcare facility and vocational education at a university under one program. During this period (1997–2016), thanks to support from the Dutch government, there have been great strides in the development of the advanced practitioner nursing profession.

In 2004, the Dutch government underlined the importance of this profession by making grants available for salary compensation and compensation for training on the hospital ward for these professionals. To qualify for these compensation possibilities, the college and healthcare institutions must work together formally. The healthcare organizations became formally the employer of the NP student for the duration of the program (i.e., for a period of 2 years). The organization must employ a physician and/or an NP as practical educators on the ward. In addition, they must write a job-function-profile for the tasks the NP student should perform after finishing the education so that the organization and the NP student know which tasks are expected of them after finishing their study. This job-function-profile covers the Dutch NP competencies.

In 2009, legislation was developed to guarantee the quality of education and work for NPs. The following requirements were formulated:

- Regulations that universities and employers must follow when educating NP students
- Regulations that a student graduate must follow to register in the Dutch NP registry to be licensed
- Regulations on how many accreditation-points a NP must collect yearly to maintain registration (NPs must re-register every 5 years)
- Regulation for title protection (the Dutch title is "Nurse Specialist")
- The specialty that the NP could choose from. These specialties include the following domains:
  1. Somatic care prevention
  2. Somatic acute care
  3. Somatic intensive care
  4. Chronic somatic care
  5. Mental health

The selection of a specialty must be based on the nature of their work respectively: prevention and identification of healthcare risks; prevention and treatment of acute healthcare problems; treatment of somatic health problems; ongoing treatment of the medical condition; tertiary prevention; coping with impairments, disabilities, and handicaps resulting from one or more chronic somatic disorders (comorbidity); social inclusion; and treatment of mental health problems. Nurse practitioners specialized in domain 2 or 3 work more from a medical point of view, therefore, the "International Classification of Diseases" forms a central element in their clinical reasoning. Nurse Practitioners specialized in domain 4 work more from a nursing perspective, therefore, the "International Classification of Human Functioning" forms the central element for their clinical reasoning. Nurse Practitioners specialized in domain 5 focused on mental health issues use the "Diagnostic and Statistical Manual of Mental Disorders" as their basis.

In 2011, the Dutch government enriched the Dutch Individual Healthcare Professions Act (IHCP Act, in Dutch Wet BIG) with an addition to this act that provided NP direct authorization to perform, without interference of physicians, a set of procedures that pose unacceptable health risks to patients if performed by individuals with insufficient professional competence. These procedures are called "reserved procedures" and include: (1) the performance of low complex minor surgical actions, (2) the performance of catheterization, (3) giving injections, (4) performing punctures, (5) the prescription of upper respiratory drugs, (6) performing elective cardioversion, (7) application of defibrillation, and (8) performing endoscopies. A 2015 evaluation demonstrated that the "reserved procedures" 1 – 5 were carried out frequently by NPs. In contrast, the "reserved procedures" 6-8 were performed less frequently. Only a small group of NPs working in cardiac care employed these interventions.

Ten universities of applied sciences in the Netherlands offer an NP education program. In close collaboration, the universities have developed a competency based program. These competencies, seven in total, are taken from the CANMEDS Physician Competency Framework [33], a framework that identifies and describes the abilities required of physicians to effectively meet the healthcare needs of the population they serve. These abilities are grouped thematically under seven roles and are housed in three internationally recognized areas of responsibility for the NP: patient care, nursing leadership and professionalism [58]. As these competencies are not all directly visible, they are translated into critical professional activities, such as direct observation of the interaction between NP students and patients, medical record review, chart simulated recall, case report review, treatment plan review, multisource feedback, objective structured clinical exam (OSCE) or direct observation of procedural skills (Mini CEX) [63, 124].

Nearly 20 years after the introduction of the NP role in the Netherlands, a total of 2750 NPs have been educated and registered. NPs are not only seen as a substitution for medical tasks, but also for additional tasks aimed at improving and streamlining patient care. Most of the time, NPs work within the direct patient care (±80 % of their time). They fulfill the role of clinician and integrate medical and nursing clinical reasoning. From this perspective they take care of patients with a focus on human functioning, not solely on disease management. Their core tasks are focused on the organization of care and the support for patients and their families (including self-management, coping with disease).

In general, the patient population is most of the time restricted to a medical sub-specialty, such as oncology (e.g., breast cancer care), cardiac care, clinical gastroen-terology, hepatology, geriatric, psychiatry (e.g., addictions and mood disorders), mentally disabled, or primary healthcare. Nurse practitioners, however, working in general practice and in acute medical care have a more diverse medical patient pop-ulation. Within the indirect care (±20 % of their time) NPs are responsible for the development of integrated care programs, quality improvement programs, develop-ing protocols/guidelines, and promoting expertise of nurses or other caregivers. (J. Peters, HAN University of Applied Sciences, Nijmegen, the Netherlands, 17 February 2016, personal communication)

2.2.3.2 The United Kingdom: Easing the Workload of General Practitioners

Advanced nurse practitioner (ANP) roles have evolved throughout the United Kingdom for over 30 years. ANPs were initially employed in general practitioner (GP) surgeries to ease the workload of the GP. There has been an increase in num-bers over the years with the ANPs carving out their roles by developing specialist interests and becoming business partners in primary care practices. Emergency and urgent care departments have also seen more ANPs employed due to the high num-ber of patients presenting with minor injuries and minor ailments in addition to patients presenting with undifferentiated and undiagnosed conditions. Advanced nurse practitioners have undertaken a variety of functions such as night practitioners in acute hospital settings, surgical practitioners in theaters, community matrons, and primary care nurse practitioners.

Competencies for advanced practice have been delineated and published by the Royal College of Nursing [113] and endorsed by the Nursing and Midwifery Council (NMC). Even though ANPs have become integral to healthcare delivery, debate continues regarding educational standards, use of title, and regulation of the profession. Changes in health policies have also influenced educational programs provided by the National Health Service (NHS) and Higher Education Institutions. The RCN [113] guidelines advise nurses wishing to be advanced nurse practitioners to undertake RCN accredited advanced nurse practitioner educational programs as a "quality kite mark" indicating proper preparation and competence in the role.

Nurse prescribing has been a turbulent undertaking in the UK and not necessarily aligned with ANP. To prescribe a medicine or medicinal product, the nurse pre-scriber must be registered with the NMC, have undertaken appropriate training, and granted authorization/license to prescribe from the formulary that is linked to their recordable qualification. Since 2006, independent and supplementary non-medical prescribers in the UK have been able to prescribe freely for any medical condition within their scope of practice and competence with the exception of certain con-trolled drugs. Since May 2012, this right has been extended to include British National Formulary (BNF) schedule 2-5 controlled drugs. The National Prescribing Centre (NPC) has also developed a competency framework for nonmedical pre-scribers, and many of the NPC competencies can be aligned with those of the RCN and NMC in relation to advanced clinical practice.

A critical issue with advanced practice nursing from a UK perspective is that there is more focus on interprofessional practice and education, i.e., curriculum and credentialing aimed towards advanced clinical practice – comprising nurses and allied health professionals (mainly paramedics and physiotherapists). This is particularly evident in the advanced critical care practitioner (ACCP) and the emergency advanced clinical practitioner (EACP) curricula. In addition, both of these are medically led curricula mapped against registrar training for anesthetics and emergency care respectively. The recent change of name by the AANPEUK (Association of Advanced Nursing Practice Educators UK) to AAPEUK (Association of Advanced Practice Educators UK) is reflective of this move.

The exception at the moment is the ANP proposed curriculum in general practice that has been designed exclusively for nurses and, although mapped against the general practitioner curriculum, it has been nurse led. However, based on a recent government paper [59], primary care advanced practice is likely to change too and may soon resemble the interprofessional education/multiprofessional workforce seen in emergency and critical care. There are proposals (some already implemented) for paramedics, physician associates, nurse practitioners, and pharmacists to take some of the roles currently being done by general practitioners in line with restructuring of primary care services [129], (S. Sibanda, 11 February 2016, personal communication). (This section provides a comprehensive overview of the situation in the United Kingdom. See individual profiles of the four UK nations (England, Northern Ireland, Scotland, Wales) in Sect. 2.4.1.6).

2.2.4   Legislation, Policy, Healthcare Reform Promoting Momentum

Changes in legislation, policy, and healthcare reform are identified as impacting momentum when advanced practice nurses are introduced as one healthcare professional category in the healthcare workforce. Australia, People's Republic of China, and Finland provide illustrations of this perspective.

2.2.4.1 Australia: A Healthcare Workforce Perspective

The Australian healthcare system is a complex web of federal, state and territory funding, and responsibilities. As a federated nation of six states and two territories, there is no single overarching "healthcare system," rather, all levels of government—the Commonwealth, the states, and territories, as well as local government—share responsibility for health. They have different roles (funders, policy developers, regulators, and service deliverers) and in many cases those roles are shared. This division of responsibility is also a feature of the education, training, and employment of healthcare professionals. Along with the Commonwealth and state and territory governments, private employers, universities, vocational education providers, professional registration boards, and specialist colleges all have some capacity to influence the education, registration, and employment pathways of the healthcare workforce. Partnership and collaboration is therefore fundamental to the functioning of the system and achievement of any reform.

The healthcare workforce in Australia covers many occupations, ranging from highly qualified professionals to support staff and volunteers. Around 70% or $25 billion a year of recurrent hospital expenditure goes to the healthcare workforce.[1] Like many countries, the healthcare needs of the population have shifted from a focus on acute services to the management of chronic conditions that require a focus on prevention as the population ages. Reducing inefficiency in the health system and increasing its financial sustainability in the long term requires reorganization of health services, professionals and health practitioners and their associated scope of practice.

On 1 July 2010, Australia introduced a National Registration and Accreditation Scheme (NRAS) for healthcare professionals. Fourteen professional groups are covered under this scheme. The Nursing and Midwifery Board of Australia (NMBA) is responsible for the registration and accreditation of nurses and midwives under the NRAS.

Nursing in Australia includes registered nurses (RN), enrolled nurses (EN), and nurse practitioners (NP). RNs, ENs, and NPs are regulated by the NMBA. Assistants in nursing (AINs), while not part of the regulated nursing profession, have a key role in patient care in residential aged care and increasingly in the acute hospital setting.

In September 2015[2] there were:

- 261,582 practicing registered RNs in Australia.
- 1287 endorsed NPs, comprising a small but increasing component of the workforce. 80% of NPs are female and their median age is 49. The most frequent area of practice (22%) is emergency and 60% of NPs work in hospitals.
- 59,160 practicing ENs. ENs are required to work under the direct or indirect supervision of the RN.
- As members of the nursing support workforce, AINs provide limited patient care under the supervision of RNs and the direction of RNs and ENs. AINs do not have minimum mandated educational requirements.

Nurse practitioners must practice within the regulatory framework established by the NMBA including the Nurse Practitioner Standards for Practice, Code of Ethics, Code of Professional Conduct, Professional Boundaries, Continuing Professional Development, and Recency of Practice.

There are various other roles that nurses may perform at an advanced level for all or part of their practice. These vary by employer and jurisdiction and are not formally recognized by the NMBA. As mentioned, currently the majority of NPs are employed in the acute sector and tend to focus in specialty areas (e.g., emergency), but as services move to a greater primary healthcare focus there will be an

---

[1] Duckett et al. [47].

[2] http://www.nursingmidwiferyboard.gov.au/About/Statistics.aspx. Accessed 18 February 2016.

increasing need for NPs who can work broadly within primary healthcare services and models. This provides opportunities for improved utilization of these nurses and their knowledge and skills. (K. Cook, Health Workforce Division & D. Thoms, Chief Nursing and Midwifery Officer – Australian Government Department of Health, 18 February 2016, personal communication)

2.2.4.2 People's Republic of China: Assessing the Landscape for Advanced Nursing Practice

Consultants from Australia and the United States presented a landscaping report to the China Medical Board China Nursing Network (CCNN) in 2015 for the development of the Chinese Advanced Nursing Practice Program. The report set out a number of recommendations regarding the development of standards for advanced practice nursing (APN), the development of curricula for clinical/professional Master of Nursing Program based on the standards, issues surrounding the implementation of pilot projects, the educational preparation of Specialty Nurses (SN) to participate in the pilot projects and the need to establish terms of reference for committees overseeing the project. An action plan setting out key activities was undertaken to bring this project forward [62].

CCNN planned an Advanced Nursing Practice Program in PR China from May 2015 to May 2017, focusing on the education and career development pathway of advanced practice nurses (APNs). As nursing in PR China is currently transitioning towards professionalization, the need for APNs with postgraduate education qualifications is an important component of this development. In 2014, the Chinese Ministry of Education (MOE) approved 58 new clinical/professional Master of Nursing Programs. This means there will be more clinical nurses with a master's degree. Priorities for Chinese nursing are:

1. To develop a clinical career ladder system for APNs.
2. To build a specialty nurse accreditation system and practice model.
3. To expand the SN nursing role from hospital to community.

The Advanced Nursing Practice Program is being initiated to contribute to these three priority areas. A Chinese Advanced Nursing Practice Program Executive Committee comprised of Nursing Deans from Fudan University, Peking Union Medical College and Peking University and Nursing Directors from affiliated hospitals has been established to facilitate this process. Two overseas nursing professors from Johns Hopkins University, USA, and from The University of Melbourne, Australia, served as advisors to this program. They provided advice to the Executive Committee on strategic directions and actions for establishing the Advanced Nursing Practice Program [62].

Advanced practice roles are informally being implemented across PR China in recognition of the need to expand the scope of nursing practice to meet changing population and healthcare delivery needs. Noting this situation, the Chinese Government has given approval for clinical/professional degrees at master's level aimed at training nurses to develop advanced practice competencies. By 2011, 28 universities in PR China had recruited nursing students into clinical/professional degree programs in various clinical areas indicating a new developmental phase in graduate nursing education in PR China. In 2014, 58 new clinical/professional masters programs were approved. The total number of clinical/professional master's program in nursing reached 84 by the end of March 2015 in China. This development for nursing is in line with the Central Government's 10-year plan to increase clinical training of physicians. The CCNN wants nursing to also plan for greater clinical experience and specialist training, ensuring, where possible, that nursing stays in parallel with medicine in terms of experience and advanced training for specialty practice.

Even though the China Medical Board China Nursing Network has one focus on nursing education for ANP, the starting point for the scheme is a comprehensive and policy based approach. Taking into account unofficial progression of extended nursing practice in place and in consultation with external experts, an overall plan of action has been proposed. (M. Hill, Johns Hopkins University, USA, 20 January 2016, personal communication)

2.2.4.3 Finland: A Newly Launched Advanced Nursing Practice Initiative Consistent with Social and Healthcare Reform

The concept of APN has not been traditionally used in Finland, but there are nurses working in various advanced clinical roles, as well as in primary healthcare and in hospitals. Finland has a long experience of close cooperation and task sharing between physicians and nurses, especially in primary care centers. Advanced roles for registered nurses have been developed more systemically since the early 2000s, e.g., the first CNSs (clinical nurse specialist) appeared at that time and more are coming on to the professional scene. Nurses' limited right to prescribe medicines was introduced in 2010. Nevertheless, the APN is still at a relatively early developmental phase in Finland.

The Finnish Nurses Association nominated a group of experts in 2013 to examine the current situation of APN in Finland and to give recommendations and grounds for further developmental work. The report by the group was officially launched on 11 April 2016. The report suggests to introduce two roles: clinical nurse specialist (CNS) and nurse practitioner (NP), with Finnish translations for the titles. The Finnish clinical career path for nurses in the advanced roles is described based on the international literature and adapted to national standards and needs. The report includes five recommendations: (1) establish coherent titles, defined job descriptions and legislative changes, (2) establish education programs/access to education to ensure the APNs obtain the required competencies (3) identify the number of APN nurses needed in the country based on the population's healthcare needs, (4) ensure that wages correlate to the responsibilities and duties of the work, and (5) define a system to evaluate and follow the effectiveness and outcomes of the roles.

At the launching event, the audience of approximately 40 people, including representatives from the Ministry of Culture and Education; Ministry of Social Affairs and Health; the National Supervisory Authority for Welfare and Health and the

President of the Finnish Medical Association, were present. There was a vibrant and constructive discussion between all the stakeholders with positive support especially from both ministries to continue the work of establishing the APN roles. The pioneers of this initiative are persevering relentlessly.

It is anticipated that the next event will be a seminar in the fall of 2016 to gather key stakeholders to discuss education, implementation, and additional strategies to promote the APN roles. The momentum for the introduction of APN in Finland currently is the significant social and healthcare reform that is about to take place. The anticipated effects of the APN roles are consistent with the main aim of the reform: to decrease inequity of social and health services, to promote accurate access to care, to facilitate accessible healthcare service paths for patients and to improve the management of healthcare costs. (A. Suutaria, Head of International Affairs, Finnish Nurses Association, 11 May 2016, personal communication)

2.2.5 Enhancing the Status of Nursing: A Career Incentive

The ANP concept offers nurses an incentive to remain in the profession and continue to practice in an advanced clinical capacity. The attraction of the APN roles has the potential of appealing to future students as well as to encourage current nurses to choose an advanced clinical career path. Singapore and Hong Kong present illustrations of this motivation.

2.2.5.1 Singapore: Professional Potential in Clinical Nursing

Impetus for the APN role in Singapore is attributed to a plea by nursing and nursing leaders for clinical career advancement along with a view that nurses with advanced skills and knowledge could fill gaps and add quality in the provision of healthcare services [121]. Historically, Singapore had been losing highly skilled nurses to management and education career tracks for promotion and remuneration. Key decision makers envisioned that creation of a clinical career path would retain nurses in clinical practice and enhance the status of nursing in the country [7]. Noting this situation, formal and informal discussions among nursing leaders and key stakeholders provided the conceptual beginnings for ANP in Singapore.

In 1997, a national Nursing Task Force recommended implementation of a nurse clinician role to keep highly skilled nurses in clinical practice [82]. A hybrid model based on the clinical nurse specialist and nurse practitioner roles observed in the United States provided the foundation for the Singapore APN role [73]. The initial academic program was introduced at the National University of Singapore (NUS) in January 2003 under the auspices of the Yong Loo Lin School of Medicine and is now managed under the direction of the Alice Lee Centre of Nursing Studies. The use of the title "Advanced Practice Nurse" is protected under the Amendment to the Singapore Nurses' and Midwives' Act that was passed in 2005 [98]. These regulations include a role definition, scope of practice, and role competencies based on the ICN recommendations [65].

The Ministry of Health (MOH) has been pivotal to the feasibility and sustainability of the APN initiative. Unlike countries where candidates for education programs are self-funded and the potential students independently choose their university or education program, all student fees are fully funded by the Singapore MOH. An employer (hospital, polyclinic, or other healthcare institution) selects the potential candidate from the current nursing staff and the employing institution pays a full salary during the period that the nurse is a student. The nurses agree to fulfill a bonding period for 2–3 years following graduation and successful completion of their APN internship. Upon successful completion of the Master of Nursing (MN) degree at NUS, the APN graduate must complete a minimum of a one-year supervised internship in order to qualify for certification, registration, and licensure as an APN. Since the entrance of the first students into the master's program in 2003, the number of APN students has grown from 15 in the initial cohort to annual intakes of 20 – 25 students. As of September 2016, 172 students had completed the APN program and were in clinical practice.

The majority of APNs are in hospital-based settings ranging from intensive care units, heart failure clinics, preoperative services, and mental health specialties. A decision was made in 2012 to include pediatrics in the academic curriculum. The Singaporean national healthcare agenda has developed an increased focus on chronic illness and mental health needs, especially as they relate to the aging population. As a result, the MOH has envisioned that more services should be accessible in the community. The anticipation of increased demands on the health systems in the country and a shortage of physicians in certain specialties provide additional momentum supporting a call for more APNs in various healthcare settings.

The path to successful role implementation was uncertain at times when attempting to differentiate what the APN can do that is different from the generalist nurse or the nurse clinicians who already held positions of advanced responsibility in the Singapore healthcare systems. A career ladder with a clinical path was established in the initial phase of APN development; however, at first it was difficult for APNs to receive promotion if their focus was clinical practice. Medical staff and nurse managers were puzzled initially over the position and function of APNs in the healthcare workforce. However, as the roles have evolved key stakeholders, nursing leaders, nurses themselves, and additional healthcare providers share a sense of pride in the increased status and professional development for nursing that has accompanied academic education for the APN roles [108, 121, 123].

2.2.5.2 Hong Kong: Career Advancement

Similarly, in Hong Kong the consideration of advanced practice nursing roles was viewed as career advancement and promotion for nurses. Advanced practice nurses began as nurse specialists (NS) in Hong Kong in 1994 followed by the introduction of the "umbrella" title APN in 2003 [127]. The Hospital Authority introduced the position of nurse consultant (NC) into the Nurses Career Structure and Progression Model in 2009 with the primary aim to broaden the nursing clinical career path [79]. Under this structure, a registered nurse can progress to APN and NC in a specific clinical field. The Hospital Authority is not a regulatory agency but manages all the public hospitals and covers about 80 % of in-patient hospital services in Hong Kong.

The suggested requirements of an NC are in four main areas: academic, research, clinical, and leadership competency. An NC is required to have at least a master's degree in clinical streams of nursing, have completed nursing specialty training, general education in other specialties and be able to track specialty educational planning and teaching experiences. In addition, an NC is expected to have at least 8 years of specialty clinical experience, preferably in advanced roles and demonstrate specialty expert clinical skills and care innovations. Evidence of leadership and management skills with cross-specialty and inter-professional working experiences are advantageous for becoming an NC. The first NCs were appointed in five clinical specialties: diabetes, renal, wound, and stoma care, psychiatrics, and continence and were appointed to seven different specialty units in Hong Kong public hospitals [79]. A study done by Lee et al. [79] demonstrated that the introduction of the NC is enhancing quality of healthcare services in Hong Kong.

Prior to introduction of the NC, Hong Kong Hospital Authority had introduced nurse led clinics with NSs directing service provision. The NS often carries their own patient load and may see patients on other hospital wards that have specialty needs. The role of these specialists within the hospital systems varies according to hospital and specialty [36]. The presence of the NS preceded the NC concept with experience as an NS included in the criteria to become an NC in this career advancement scheme.

Hong Kong's healthcare system does not have a significant presence of primary healthcare services, thus individuals are usually seen for a significant ailment in the emergency department. Once diagnosed and stabilized within the hospital setting, patients will then be referred to an outpatient specialty clinic. Due to the limited number of these clinics, the Hospital Authority developed the concept of nurse-led clinics with specialty nurses providing care and management to a specific population [36]. Since inception, these nurse-led clinics, managed by NSs, have continued to expand and demonstrate improvement to the healthcare services in Hong Kong. It is estimated that the NS in these nurse led clinics can manage up to 90 % of patients for outpatient disease-specific care [128].

This section has identified four drivers that stimulated interest in launching ANP initiatives and linked country profiles to each incentive to demonstrate the diversity of rationale associated with the inclusion of advanced nursing roles. These exemplars and the country profiles that follow in Sect. 2.4 portray how multifaceted and complex the impetus for advanced nursing initiatives can be. Launching an ANP scheme and introducing the concept can be a coming together of more than one driver with support from national and international organizations. The next section discusses how international assistance and encouragement can be helpful.

2.3   International Influence

Building on earlier content in this chapter the following sections highlight the influence international organizations can exert in promoting the ANP concept. International organizations can provide the authority and support an initiative may need to convince key stakeholders and healthcare decision makers of the benefits of advanced nursing practice. When a scheme is viewed as part of global advancement for nursing versus only a local or national directive, this backing offers an increased level of credibility for consideration of the concept. Sections 2.3.1, 2.3.2, and 2.3.3 describe how three international organizations support and promote the advancement of nursing practice.

2.3.1   ICN (International Council of Nurses)

Noting the growth of ANP globally, ICN launched the International Nurse Practitioner/Advanced Practice Nursing Network (INP/APNN) in 2000 to provide organizational support and to follow trends and new developments in the field. This network has acted as a resource for the international nursing and healthcare community by providing and disseminating information on ANP. Network activities have been facilitated by biennial conferences, biannual news bulletins and ongoing research projects. News and reports have been posted on the network website: http://www.icn-apnetwork.org

The key goal of the ICN Network has been an international resource for nurses practicing in nurse practitioner (NP) or advanced practice nursing (APN) roles, and interested others (e.g., policymakers, educators, regulators, health planners) by:

- Making relevant and timely information about practice, education, role development, research, policy and regulatory developments, and appropriate events widely available
- Providing a forum for sharing and exchange of knowledge expertise and experience
- Supporting nurses and countries who are in the process of introducing or developing NP or APN roles and practice
- Accessing international resources that are pertinent to this field (accessed 16 February 2016 from http://www.icn-apnetwork.org)

In addition, ICN through the expertise of members of the INP/APN Network developed international guidelines for a definition, scope of practice, standards and competencies for advanced nursing practice to promote role development and facilitate multinational research [65]. The decision by ICN to take an official position on nurse practitioner and advanced nursing roles provides a benchmark from which member countries and others can utilize the definitive information and adapt pertinent sections for country specific initiatives (see Sect. 1.1 for the ICN definition and characteristics of the advanced practice nurse).

The International Council of Nurses also actively represents nursing in such global arenas as the World Health Organization's governing body, the World Health Assembly, and provides representation to additional international organizations to ensure that nursing is visible in discussions of cost effective and quality healthcare programs for the world's populations. In July 2016, after 16 years of focusing attention on international ANP development through the INP/APN Network and a change in ICN administrative policies, the International Council of Nurses is reviewing the functionality of their nine networks including the INP/APNN. A change in ICN infrastructure will continue to support the advancement of nursing within a new organizational model. The ICN website is http://www.icn.ch.

2.3.2   IFNA (International Federation of Nurse Anesthetists)

The International Federation of Nurse Anesthetists (IFNA) is a global organization representing nurse anesthetists. IFNA was founded in 1989 with eleven charter members: Austria, Germany, Finland, France, Iceland, Norway, Sweden, South Korea, Switzerland, United States and the former Yugoslavia. This international organization is dedicated to advancing global education and practice standards in order to promote the art, science, and safety of anesthesia care. The IFNA has 40 country members and is managed by a board of Country National Representatives (CNRs). Country membership in IFNA stipulates that the applicant organization is the country's most representative national nurse anesthetist association. A Country National Representative (CNR) serves on the IFNA board and is the liaison back to the country. Non-nursing associations and anesthesia technicians that are not nurses may join IFNA as associate members.

Nurses have been providing anesthesia care worldwide for over 150 years. A survey by McAuliffe and Henry [84] confirmed that nurses provide anesthesia services in 107 countries. The IFNA provides the definition of a nurse anesthetist as a person who has completed a program of basic nursing education plus basic nurse anesthesia education and is qualified/authorized in his or her country to practice nurse anesthesia. While the names or titles of nurses administering anesthesia vary globally, a nurse anesthetist is an advanced practice nurse who provides or participates in the provision of advanced specialized nursing and anesthesia services. These services may include anesthesia and anesthesia related services such as respiratory care, cardiopulmonary resuscitation, and other emergent services.

An international accreditation program for nurse anesthesia entitled "Anesthesia Program Approval Process" (APAP) as well as a model curriculum for education programs has been developed by IFNA. There are currently 20 nurse anesthesia programs located in the following countries: China, Denmark, France, Iceland, Indonesia, Philippines, Sweden, Switzerland, the Netherlands, Tunisia, and the USA. With the success of the APAP program, IFNA is developing a framework and guidelines for a Continuous Professional Development (CPD) program.

IFNA has also assisted countries in the development of the specialty of nurse anesthesia. In Indonesia, for example, IFNA assisted the country in curriculum redevelopment resulting in the opening of five new nurse anesthesia programs. Japan joined IFNA in June of 2014 and immediately began working on ways to develop the Asian Society of Nurse Anesthetists (ASNA) in order to establish an association that could work cooperatively to help meet anesthesia needs within the region. The Japan CNR with IFNA assistance secured a grant to support development of the infrastructure of the ASNA. The CNRs of South Korea, Japan, Taiwan, and the USA form the research team for the ASNA grant. In November 2015, representatives of these four countries attended their third joint meeting in Kyoto, Japan to discuss their research results and prepare for report submission.

The IFNA collaboration with institutions that have a professional interest in nurse anesthesia includes: affiliate membership in ICN, membership and participation in the WHO Global Initiative for Essential and Emergency Surgical Care (WHO GIEESC), liaisons with the World Federation of Societies of Anesthesiologists (WFSA) and European Society of Anesthesiology (ESA). The IFNA is a member of the Centre for Quality Assurance in International Education (CQAIE), the International Hospital Federation (IHF) and the International Society for Quality in Healthcare (ISQua). Furthermore, the IFNA encourages its member countries to develop relationships with other professional healthcare organizations and assists member countries with policy, education, and practice information needed for promotion of the specialty of nurse anesthesia. IFNA website: http://www.ifna-int.org/ifna/news.php. (J. Rowles, IFNA President, 07 February 2016, personal communication)

2.3.3 WHO (World Health Organization)

As an agency of the United Nations, WHO works to further international cooperation aimed at improving health conditions worldwide. The approach of WHO is not specific to nursing but it can influence the extent of attention given to nursing professionals and their presence in provision of healthcare services. By taking a leading role in encouraging governments to deal with emergent healthcare issues, WHO acts as a mechanism for providing attention and debate over the need for restructuring and more effective inclusion of nursing and midwifery services. The organization works with a broad range of partners at the global, regional, and country levels in efforts to promote strengthening nursing and midwifery services including advanced nursing practice [148].

WHO activities occur more directly under the guidance of its regional offices and Regional Directors of Nursing. For example, in 2000 the WHO Regional Nursing Director for the Eastern Mediterranean Region (EMRO) supported a proactive position to promote exploration and support for advanced nursing practice in the region. In 2001, 14 member nations of EMRO gathered in Pakistan to discuss, explore, and offer recommendations for establishing advanced nursing practice and nurse prescribing [149]. An action plan and supportive documents were shaped as a result. Following the 2001 regional WHO meeting, representatives of the Sultanate of Oman and the Kingdom of Bahrain, member nations of EMRO, with support from WHO regional office commenced to investigate the possibility of advanced nursing roles in their respective countries [119, 120]. Subsequently and with continued WHO regional support, the Sultanate of Oman proceeded to develop a framework for the possibility of introducing advanced nursing roles [1]. If successful, Oman has the possibility of providing an ANP model for the rest of the region. The Omani situation exemplifies one type of international organizational support that encouraged progression of interest in the ANP concept over a period of time from 2001 to 2016 (see Sect. 2.4.6 for the Oman country profile).

When effective, international organizations provide the capacity to strengthen support for advanced nursing practice by conducting discussion forums, organizing conferences, sharing information through publications, and providing consultancy expertise. Resources, evidence, and support from an international platform can incentivize groups and key decision makers to consider country specific proposals. The next section presents additional examples of how a variety of countries explored and developed advanced nursing schemes.

2.4   Country Profiles

The country specific profiles in this section reveal the complexities of introducing new nursing roles into the healthcare workforce and underline the diversity in which these roles become part of the cadre of healthcare professionals. There does not appear to be one common starting point when commencing with an ANP initiative, instead, it is the diversity in bringing together varied interests that is striking. Roles may evolve in response to a healthcare need, as a country scheme to enhance service delivery or as a plan to promote an advanced professional nursing identity (see Sect. 2.1 for further discussion of incentives and motivation for ANP).

There is extensive academic rhetoric attempting to define, describe, identify, and even oppose the phenomenon of ANP. Views posed when referring to the ANP concept range from passionate support to rigid resistance. It is the intent of the author that the country profiles portrayed in this chapter and in other sections of this publication are regarded as illustrations of development that could be used by healthcare planners and decision makers according to their own country inclinations and capacity. A descriptive or narrative style of country cases from national representatives has, in most instances, been followed in providing country specific details. The author has adhered to this format in order to respectively portray country development from the perspective of the international sources. Country narratives illustrate the range of development worldwide but are not intended to represent the entirety of international interest. In addition, the author acknowledges that different country representatives might provide another perspective of national development. In addition, every effort has been made to maintain the accuracy of the country profiles as provided by the contributors. Minor editing has been done only to aid the reader in understanding the provided information.

2.4.1   Europe: Significant Advanced Nursing Practice Growth

Regional support in addition to international influence can attract attention for the consideration and development of ANP. Although many initiatives in Europe are in their infancy, there has been significant escalation in the Region. The following sections provide country profiles representing this increase.

2.4.1.1 European Federation of Nurses Association Involvement Contributes to Advanced Practice Nursing in Europe

The European Federation of Nurses Association (EFN) was established in 1971 to represent the nursing profession and its interests to the European Institutions, based on the nursing education and free movement Directives being drafted by the European Commission at that time. The EFN is the independent voice of more than three million nurses over 34 National Nurses Associations (NNA), Regulators or Unions at European Level.

More intensive work for advanced practice nursing (APN) started in 2011 at EFN when the beginning of the modernization of Directive 2005/36/EC started with an EU Public Consultation that brought upfront the challenges faced in the recognition process and the need to update the undergraduate education requirements of the professions covered under the automatic systems. It was clear that the content of nurse education of the Directive needed to be updated to reflect current advancements in nursing such as new focus of healthcare oriented towards prevention, long-term care, community-based care, eHealth and ICT (information and communication technology) developments, patient safety, and research and evidence-based practice. During the modernization process, the negotiation of the Commission's proposal with the European Parliament and Council resulted in the strengthening of the nurse education requirements and the addition of a set of eight competencies. The EFN was very much involved in the elaboration of those competencies that were used during the negotiations and presented to the Parliament, Council, Commission and stakeholders during a European Parliament Roundtable on the nurse education organized by the EFN in October 2012. Once the modernized Directive 2013/55/EU was approved, the main focus of EFN went on to ensure that all these changes are being transposed into the national legislation in all Member States. This work continues with work of three categories of nursing care: general care nurse (RN), specialist nurse (SN), and advanced nurse practitioner (ANP). Definitions of these categories are in line with ICN definitions and modernized Directive 2013/55/EU [44].

Advance Practice Nursing

The increasing and changing health needs of citizens of the European Union (EU) have led to member states considering new ways of organizing and delivering health and social care. Within a context of tighter health budgets and rising demands for high quality and safe care, advanced roles for nurses are required to make best use of the resources available and enhance quality. That is why EFN had an EU project "ENS4Care" [48] which shared good nursing and social work practices in eHealth services (telehealth and telecare) and created a guideline through evaluation and consensus building focusing, e.g., on skills development for advanced roles.

In Europe, as in other regions of the world, advanced practice is a new way of delivering cost-effective care and increasing access to qualified healthcare practitioners. Advanced nurse practitioner is a registered nurse who has acquired the expert knowledge base, complex decision-making skills, and clinical competencies for expanded practice, the characteristics of which are shaped by the context and/or country in which s/he is credentialed to practice (European Federation of Nurses

Associations). Advanced roles for nurses are being developed in response to increasing and rapidly changing healthcare needs within restricted budgets [43] and are seen as the way forward to improve access to care and patient outcomes, contain provider related costs and improve recruitment and retention rates of nurses through enhanced career prospects [19, 40]. One of the fundamental pillars to promote high quality healthcare is through a highly educated, dedicated, and skilled workforce. Specifically, the promotion of advanced roles for nurses has been demonstrated to boost quality, safety, and cost-effectiveness of the healthcare delivered. These roles have made an enormous difference on the governance and management of healthcare, and improve efficiency, enhance patient care, improve health outcomes, contributing ultimately to the sustainability of health systems.

One good example of the advanced role is nurse prescribing. Nurse prescribing has made huge steps forward in the past few years and is being fully implemented in several Member States (United Kingdom, Ireland, Finland, Sweden, Spain). Nurse prescribing is one of the guidelines based on identified best practice examples collected through the ENS4Care [49] network and as such is rooted in the daily practice experience of nurses and social workers. Evidence suggests that this implementation is safe and clinically appropriate [6, 78, 145], and shows that nurse prescribing improves patient care by ensuring timely access to medicines and treatment and increasing flexibility for patients [34, 46, 93]. Nurse prescribing is first and foremost about making a difference for patients and service users. It is about enhancing professional capacity and developing new skills that lead to services that are more patient-focused thereby delivering better outcomes.

New technology, eHealth and associated professional advances are becoming increasingly important for delivering high quality care to all European citizens. Therefore, the modernized European Union Directive 55, especially article 31 on nurses' competencies, is key to strengthening the nursing workforce and as such support also the RN4cast findings [2, 50]. (M. Sipilä, President EFN, 28 April 2016, personal communication)

2.4.1.2 The Introduction of Advanced Nursing Practice in the French Health System

Increase in life expectancy, high incidence of chronic diseases[3] combined with a physician shortage in France, created difficulties for health consumers to get access to the healthcare they need where they live. In a growing number of regions in France, people have to wait many months to get a medical appointment or they go to the emergency department to treat minor ailments. A new concept appeared in France: « medical deserts » to describe these territories where finding a physician is a challenge. The reduction of the hospital length of stay and the cuts made in hospital staff modify their practices and organization. Even though needs are high, not enough time is dedicated to patient education, integration, and coordination of complex care paths and coordination. Illness prevention and health education, which

---

[3] In 2007, around 15 million patients are living with chronic diseases in France. DGS plan 2007–2011.

promote change in risk behaviors, still need to be improved in France. Definitively, a paradigm change is needed in the healthcare system to promote a more wholistic approach to patients and family.[4] Only patient centered care would improve clinical outcomes, well being, and quality of life. Many countries encounter the same difficulties and some of them develop strategies to cope adequately with this situation. Advanced nursing practice represents one of these strategies whose efficacy has been demonstrated in many impact studies.[5]

Advanced Nursing Practice Officially Introduced in France: A Decision After Years of Discussions

After years of discussion, an article introducing advanced practice in nursing and allied health professions (AHP) in France was inserted in a public health law voted by the French parliament in January 2016.[6] The nurse practitioner profile seems to have been preferred. This decision now needs to be implemented, but many operational aspects of this implementation process are still to be written.

Nurses are concerned by this reform. France is not beginning from scratch in this field. Since the 1990s, postregistration programs dedicated to developing clinical experts in nursing were introduced in France by private educational non-academic institutions: "Certified nurse clinician" (CCN) and later "certified clinical nurse specialist" (CNS) courses were available to French nurses. A growing number of these experts in nursing were certified. The competencies of these experts were fully used in clinical settings: CCN and CNS helped to improve nursing care in oncology, palliative care, pain treatment, and psychosocial care. Some of them ran consultation in different specialized fields. In many places they are considered as resource persons by patients and co-workers. Unfortunately, the added value these expert nurses bring to the healthcare system was never fully recognized in the French nurse practice act.[7] [8]

Since the beginning of the millennium, public health decision makers tried to find out solutions to counterbalance the medical shortage France in facing. Access to the medical profession is strictly regulated in France and only a small number of students are admitted to medical schools each year. Moreover, French physicians prefer working as a specialist rather than a general practitioner and work in big cities rather than in rural areas. At the end of their medical studies they can freely choose where they want to practice even if their education at medical school was highly covered by public money.

The Dean of the Medical School of Marseille published a report in 2003 exploring this issue. His recommendation was to allow healthcare professionals to collaborate in a different way allowing nurses and AHP (Allied Health Professionals)

---

[4] Borgès Da Silva [15].

[5] Bryant-Lukosius [16].

[6] Law n° 2016-41 "modernizing our health system" voted on January 26th 2016, published in OJ N°22 January 27th 2016.

[7] Debout [37].

[8] Gic REPASI [56].

to perform medical interventions. He described this strategy as a way to provide other career pathways to nurses and AHP. For the first time in France, the concept of advanced nursing practice was mentioned in an official report.[9] Following the publication of this report, some experiments of "task delegation" between physicians and nurses/AHP were launched under the auspice of the French National Health Authority (Haute Autorité de Santé).[10]

At the same time, nursing education underwent a profound reformation in France. In 2009, a bachelor degree became the only way to enter the nursing profession. Following the recommendation made in the 2003 report and without any change made in the nursing act, two universities (Ecole des Hautes Etudes en Santé Publique and the University of Marseille) decided to set up the first master's degree program in clinical nursing practice dedicated to prepare future advanced practice nurses. The University of St Quentin-en-Yvelines launched a second program a couple of months later. These programs adopted ICN's standards in the matter of APN education and tried to adapt them to the French context. Several nursing specialties are available: oncology, gerontology, complex care coordination, chronic diseases, pain treatment/palliative care, and mental health. In 2016, about 106 nurses have graduated from this master's program in clinical nursing in France.

Advanced Practice Nurses Already Graduated in France: The Difficulties of Role Implementation

The newly graduated APNs were prepared to implement the five roles classically devoted to this category of nurses: expert clinical practice, consultation, education, leadership, and research. Their postgraduate education helped them develop their expertise in critical thinking and evidence-based practice. Nevertheless, having graduated did not ensure that these nurses could easily find a job in the French healthcare system corresponding to their level of preparation. The lack of appropriate legislation was the greatest difficulty they encountered. The APN roles were poorly defined in healthcare organizations and the added value they bring to the system was not rewarded in their salary. Obstacles, which hinder the implementation of APN in France, are also observed amongst healthcare professionals, in the ranks of nurses and physicians. Fear, suspicion, or rejection are the most common reactions experienced by these healthcare providers.

French APN: Profile and Role Implementation in the Future

A careful examination of the article introducing APN in the French healthcare system shows that in the mind of policy makers, the profile of this new healthcare professional will combine the characteristics of a physician assistant and those of a nurse practitioner. Indeed, the legislation mentions the interventions that will be in the scope of practice of these APNs: screening, education, and prevention, orientation of patients in complex situations. The APN will also perform clinical assessment and conclusions, technical care, and clinical tests. As part of an expansion of

---

[9] Berland [10].

[10] Henart et al. [61].

the nursing practice act,[11] APN will able to prescribe invasive testing and to renew medications. These interventions will be performed autonomously with full responsibility of the APN.

Advanced practice will likely include about 1–3 % of the French nursing population. Accredited universities will be able to deliver the APN diploma. However, as of May 2016 it is not known whether or not it will be a master's degree. To ensure security and quality of care provided by APNs, French nursing organizations advise the policy makers to adopt the definition of ICN [6] which recommends *a minimum* master's degree for practice as an APN.

At first sight it seems that France is moving a step forward regarding advanced nursing practice to adequately respond to health needs of its population. Although, as nurses, we must develop strategic planning and political influence in order to introduce APN in an appropriate way. As Schober et al. [123] highlighted, strategic planning at national and local level is a key to success in APN role implementation.[12] There is a need to first clarify the roles and to ensure them enough autonomy. A regulatory framework needs to be developed along with an economic model. Title protection and regulation of APN practice by the nursing regulatory body are other important issues to address as well as nursing leadership in the education of the future APN.

The law is a first step, but now nurses and APN's need to remain vigilant. The way this law will be implemented will determine how APN will be introduced in our national territory. APNs need to have full professional legitimacy and their expert skills need to be valued. The French population really needs this type of healthcare professional to improve their quality of life and equity between citizens regarding access to care. (F. Ambrosino, co coordinator, advanced nursing practice network [réseau de la pratique avancée en soins infirmiers – Gic REPASI] and C. Debout, Directeur de l'Institut de Soins Infirmiers Supérieurs, 23 March 2016, personal communication)

2.4.1.3 Advanced Nursing Practice Development in Germany

Compared to some of the developments internationally Advanced Nursing Practice (ANP) in Germany is in its infancy [80]. The expert group Sachverständigenrat zur Begutachtung der Entwicklung im Gesundheitssystem recommended for the first time in 2007 that nurses should widen their scope and practice with greater autonomy [115]. The recommendations of the expert group were echoed by stakeholders from nursing associations and from key people at higher education institutions, which paved the way for the developments in advanced nursing practice across Germany [41, 70, 115, 140, 141].

According to an evaluation undertaken by Ullmann and Lehwaldt [140] there are very few master's level programs available across Germany that prepare nurses for

---

[11] Décret n° 2004-802 du 29 juillet 2004 relatif aux parties IV et V du code de la santé publique. https://www.legifrance.gouv.fr/affichTexte.do?cidTexte=JORFTEXT000000410355&dateTexte=20040807.

[12] Schober et al. [123].

their roles in advanced practice. The existing programs could be developed through modules that have a specific focus on the development of advanced clinical competencies. Programs could also benefit from substantial practice components designed to develop APN areas of specialist practice [140]. Nurses that hold advanced clinical competencies in Germany often acquire these skills in neighboring countries such as the UK and Ireland. There are reports of nurses from Germany who gained APN clinical competencies such as, history taking and physical examination skills through designated programs and practice experiences [80, 81].

Another area that requires further development in Germany relates to legislation. What is required is a legislative framework for an advanced scope of practice and legislation that allows APNs to practice autonomously within their field [143]. Such legislation could relate to prescription rights and treatment rights. A formal system of APN licensure, registration, and credentialing, as recommended by the International Council of Nurses [65], does currently not exist in Germany as nursing boards are only beginning to form. As of May 2016, there is no legislation in place to confer and protect the title Advanced Practice Nurse. The title "Pflegeexpertin APN," which translated into English means "Nursing Expert APN" has been suggested for Germany [141]. The title has been defined by the nursing associations of the German speaking regions Deutscher Berufsverband für Pflegeberufe (DBfK), Österreichischer Gesundheits- und Krankenpflegeverband (ÖGKV), & Schweizer Berufsverband (2013) [41] based on the ICN definition of advanced practice nursing. However, without legislation to protect this title there is no consensus with regards to necessary roles and responsibilities that go with this title. There is evidence to suggest that there are highly motivated nurses in Germany, both in practice and in the areas that support advanced practice, e.g., in education and management [12, 139, 141].

Advanced nursing practice in Germany is developing from the bottom up such as shown by Teigeler [139] who reports on 17 APNs who practice at one university hospital in South Germany. The management in this hospital is committed to supporting their APNs working in direct patient care. Another role of APNs according to Teigeler [139] is practice development and staff training.

In line with their role as change agents APNs in Germany act as an intermediary between nursing science and nursing practice. This was shown in the report of another German hospital where the implementation of advanced nursing practice was described as an important part of their organizational development process based on the concept of magnet hospitals [13]. Here the APNs (titled Pflegeexperten APN in the paper) are integrated into a structure of a matrix organization, which means that they are assigned to a department, a clinical specialty, but also attend to interdepartmental tasks such as contributing to the in-house nursing education [13]. However, direct patient care remains the central aspect of the APN role in this hospital.

Publications and the records of the 2nd and 3rd International German speaking APN & ANP Congresses in Berlin (2013) and Munich (2015) show that most of the advanced practice nurses (APNs) in Germany practice in general/psychiatric adult hospital settings and in the areas of acute and chronic disease management, pediatric and community care [142, 143], as the following list demonstrates:

- Tissue viability
- Pain nurse
- Diabetes
- Breast care
- High dependency and intensive care units
- Palliative care
- Respiratory care
- Gerontology
- Psychiatry
- Delirium management and prevention
- Pediatric care
- Children and Adolescence clinics
- Dialysis therapy in children
- Working with the parents of children with tracheostomy
- Community-based oncology
- Family health
                (Decker [38], Boeckler [12], Ullmann, et al. [142, 143], Teigeler [139])

The German association Deutsches Netzwerk APN & ANP g.e.V. offers individual nurses and institutions, with an interest in developing advanced nursing roles, ongoing support through platforms for exchange and networking. The platforms that they use include regular international congresses, expert workshops and an APN Magazine. Together, nurses with an interest in APN will help to fuel the political debate and will assist in creating the necessary structures for APN in Germany. Their goal is the same, which is to enhance the patient care experience and to provide high quality autonomous direct patient care [12, 139, 141]. (D. Lehwaldt, P. Ullmann, on behalf of the board of Deutsches Netzwerk APN & ANP g.e.V., 05 May 2016, personal communication)

2.4.1.4 Advanced Nursing Practice in Iceland

The title for advanced practice in nursing in Iceland is Specialist in Nursing (SN). It is legally protected since 2003 and there is a regulation covering the requirements. The applicant must have a valid Icelandic nursing license, a master's degree in nursing and a two-year practice in nursing post-master's degree in the field he/she is seeking to be a specialist in. There is a committee evaluating the applications. However, it is not always clear what are the fields of nursing specialties. For some time medical specialization has been dominant so nurse specialist fields were, e.g., pediatric, nephrology etc. It is now acknowledged that nursing is a profession with its own specialties such as family nursing. Yet, nursing administration and patient education are not considered fields for SNs in Iceland and we wonder how to go forward with this issue.

Additional requirement for SNs' license from 2013, states that the applicant must work under the supervision of a specialist in nursing during the two-year period post-master's degree. It is not set forth in any detail how the supervision is to take place, contact hours or issues to be covered. The requirement for supervision causes frustration as it may be difficult for a new generation of specialists in nursing to claim they fulfill the requirements for a SN license. The majority of licensed SNs

(61 out of 91) work at the one university hospital in the capital city, 42 of those hold a position as a specialist within the hospital and are competent to supervise students. Of the 30 licensed SNs who do not work at the University Hospital, only four are at healthcare centers where the need for SNs is great.

At the University Hospital there is an internship program for those who have finished their master's degree and will apply for SN licensing in due time. Those enrolled use 20 % of their work time to learn about the SN role and build their career as SNs. Each intern has a support committee of three persons who assist the intern in setting forth aims and goals, ways to reach goals and assess the outcome. This program has made it possible for the University Hospital to increase the number of SNs from 25 to 44, including specialists in midwifery. In 2016 there are 15 enrolled in this program. (A. Ágústsdóttir, Project manager, Education and Research Landspitali University Hospital, Reykjavik, Iceland, 24 February 2016, personal communication)

2.4.1.5 Advanced Nurse/Midwifery Practitioner in Ireland: Twenty Years Experience

2016 marks the 20th year of Advanced Nursing/Midwifery practice in Ireland

In 1996, the concept of an emergency nurse practitioner was proposed in St James's Hospital Dublin. This initiative was intended to address a specific service need identified for patients with non-urgent clinical presentations to the Emergency Department. It was the first role of its kind in Ireland and subsequently developed across a broad range of nursing specialist areas.

As of May 2016 there are 184 registered advanced nurse/midwife (ANP/AMP) practitioners practicing at a national level within the Irish Health Service, spanning over 30 specialties. Forty-two percent of these positions operate within Emergency Departments.

One of the most fundamental changes experienced by the Irish nurses was the publication of the Commission on Nursing; A blueprint for the future, and the subsequent development of the National Council for the Professional Development of Nursing and Midwifery. The Commission on Nursing provided a unique opportunity for all Irish nurses to shape the future of clinical practice, outlining strategies to advance the nursing profession. In 1998, The Commission on Nursing recommended the establishment of a clinical career pathway leading from registration to clinical specialization and to advanced practice.

Ireland is unique in having established frameworks and standards for the expansion of nursing and midwifery roles. The process specifically emphasizes the need to involve all clinicians in the development of an ANP/AMP service and the requirement to demonstrate service need. Over the past decade Statutory Instruments have been amended to allow for the Independent Nurse prescribing of medicinal products and ionising radiation. Practice Standards as established by the Nurse Midwifery Board of Ireland have been essential to role development. Advanced nurse midwife practitioners are required to have a master's education, plus advanced medical and nurse education, specialty certification, and intensive clinical experience.

The responsibilities of the ANP/AMP extend beyond providing clinical care. The ANP/AMP is expected also to fulfill a leadership and educational role and to contribute to research and the planning and development of services.

Advanced nursing practice is concerned with harnessing the knowledge and skills of experienced nurses in the interest of better patient care and the efficient use of resources. Health Services must be run efficiently, effectively, and economically. While caring is central to the role of the ANP/AMP there is a requirement that clinical outcomes be demonstrated.

The National Council for the Professional Development of Nursing and Midwifery commissioned a joint research team from the Schools of Nursing and Midwifery, Trinity College, Dublin and the National University of Ireland, Galway to evaluate the role of the advanced nurse/midwife practitioner, focusing on the clinical and economic impact of the roles [9]. This study demonstrated conclusively that care provided by advanced nurse practitioners improves patient/client outcomes, is safe, acceptable and cost-neutral. The reality in clinical practice is that the introduction of these roles has resulted in an equitable quality patient focused service. Since the introduction of advanced practice roles there has been a marked reduction in waiting times with a reciprocal increase in patient satisfaction. Admission rates have been decreased by 50 %. Adherence to and application of international guidelines has contributed to reduced mortality and morbidity rates. Equally important, advanced practice roles have provided professional development opportunities for nurses who wish to remain in the clinical area.

Scope of Practice: Integral to Development of the Role

The Irish ANP/AMP has gone through many changes in role and regulation. We are intent on providing autonomous care to effectively meet patient/client needs. We know that in order to do this we need to challenge cultural, regulatory, and policy barriers. When the role was first introduced the prescribing of medicinal products was under supply and administration guidelines. There was no autonomy or transparency in this practice. Through partnerships and negotiations the ANP/AMP has been instrumental in contributing to changes in legislation that has resulted in independent nurse prescribing. There are still many changes pending.

The Irish Association of Advanced Nurse Practitioners was established in 2004. Membership consists of advanced nurse and midwife practitioners from a broad spectrum of specialities. Apart from the obvious benefits of peer support, creation of links and sharing of best practice, the group has been instrumental in ensuring the progression of a vision of advanced practice at both a national and international level. The ANP/AMP has integrated and become a valuable member of the multidisciplinary team. We have become integral to healthcare solutions. It is critical that all legislators know that nurse practitioners are a part of the answer to the current healthcare crisis. As advanced nurse/midwife practitioners we must also be aware of how decisions are made and how we need to participate in the decision making process. That includes getting to know the political agenda so that when a healthcare issue comes up we can direct healthcare legislation.

It's an extremely bright future. As we look to the next 20 years and beyond we remain committed to strengthening our role, working together towards the realization of our vision for advanced practice. We are on the cutting edge of nursing innovation. It is our responsibility to continue to challenge the deep-seated traditions of health professions and organizations in the interest of patient/client care. (K. Brennan, Chair, Irish Association of Advanced Nurse and Midwife Practitioners, 22 May 2016, personal communication)

2.4.1.6 United Kingdom: England, Northern Ireland, Scotland, Wales

Advanced Nursing Practice in the United Kingdom (UK) is often described as a single approach in development, however, it is helpful to take note of the differences between the four nations. Section 2.2.3.2 provides an overall perspective of the situation in the UK while this section focuses on how ANP is evolving independently in the four nations. Devolution of the United Kingdom around 2005/6 meant that each country now has a separate government. Even though the English Government theoretically has overall governing control, in reality the individual countries determine their own health policy, thus there are significant differences in philosophy and structure. For example, private healthcare providers are commonplace now in England for all types of healthcare but not in Scotland, Wales, or Northern Ireland. In Scotland and Wales prescriptions are free but in England they are not. These differences are reflected in advanced practice nursing developments. A summary of differences as related to ANP in each nation follows.

England

The Department of Health England followed Scotland and Wales in producing a position statement on Advanced Nursing, however, under the auspices of the current government this was launched as guidance thus has not really been implemented other than by educationalists using it to inform their curriculum.

This has resulted in confusion regarding what personnel call themselves and how they identify the education they have achieved. The employer governance structures have not controlled this but the perspective that a properly prepared ANP has added value for the healthcare service has been successful. As a result ANP applications supported by employers have been increasing year by year.

Health Education England has begun work on a national policy for advanced clinical practice to streamline titles, standards, and education requirements. Timelines are unclear but funding will likely follow what they develop. In 2009 England followed Scotland, Northern Ireland and Wales, and all ANP courses shifted to master's level and existing degree level courses have been phased out. Most universities admit students with prior diplomas or degrees into their master's courses if they have experience and senior nursing roles.

Northern Ireland

The Department of Health, Social Services and Public Safety in Northern Ireland (DHSSPS) through the Northern Ireland Practice and Education Council for Nursing and Midwifery (NIPEC) produced Northern Ireland's ANP framework in 2014 to provide clarity about the ANP role [97]. The Framework (p. 4):

- Provides a definition of Advanced Nursing Practice
- Highlights the associated professional support and supervision required by advanced nurse practitioners
- Identifies the core competencies and learning outcomes essential for the advanced nursing practice role
- Acts as a guide for Commissioners, workforce planners, Executive Directors of Nursing, education providers, employers, and managers of nurses, including nurses themselves.

This document emphasizes that the ANP role is clinically focused and continually evolving. In addition, components that distinguish between advanced and specialist nursing practice in the Northern Ireland context are identified.

Scotland

Under the Department of Health 2006 Modernising Nursing Careers work, NHS Executive Scotland was asked to look at advanced nursing. The Scottish Toolkit [125] was developed and was well received. However, while it discussed the need for master's level education it did not stipulate the level of the award as that of the "Advanced Nurse Practitioner" (ANP). Further work was shared arising from this situation and the Royal College of Nursing Scotland produced a document [114] showcasing the work of ANPs. The Scottish Government also made an announcement in February 2016 that includes funding of £3 million to train an additional 500 advanced nurse practitioners to bolster the skills of the profession and equip nurses across Scotland to maximize their leading role in the integrated healthcare of the future.

Wales

Wales took the lead from developments in Scotland to develop a Welsh strategy and decided to broaden the focus of the healthcare agenda to include allied health professionals and paramedics. The Chief Nursing Officer was a key driver for this work in the production of policy that is now being implemented. Interestingly, ANPs who had previously done their courses at Diploma or degree level were not grandfathered and have to do the entire master's level education and a required portfolio. No one in Wales can call themselves an advanced nurse practitioner without completing these current requirements. Organizations [employers] are struggling to release the volume of people needed for study to complete the newly regulated education requirements that are contained in this key governance framework. Due to the small scale of the Wales health service every one appears to be abiding to this change. (K. Maclaine, Course Director for Advanced Nursing Practice programs, London South Bank University, 19 February 2016, personal communication)

Sections 2.4.1.1, 2.4.1.2, 2.4.1.3, 2.4.1.4, 2.4.1.5, and 2.4.1.6 demonstrate the extent and diversity of ANP development in Europe. The following sections provide profiles of development in additional regions or countries.

2.4.2 Canada: Two Advanced Nursing Practice Roles

The Canadian Nurses Association (CNA) continues to provide leadership for the development and integration of advanced nursing practice (ANP) in Canada. In 1999, the CNA developed a framework for ANP that was revised in 2002 and 2008 [24].

Advanced nursing practice in Canada is a broad term referring to an advanced level of nursing practice that maximizes a nurse's graduate education in nursing, "in-depth nursing knowledge and expertise in meeting the health needs of individuals, families, groups, communities and populations" [24, p. 9]. There are two ANP roles in Canada: the nurse practitioner and clinical nurse specialist. Nurse practitioners are registered nurses with additional educational and experience who are able to autonomously diagnose, order and interpret tests, prescribe medications and perform specific procedures within their legislated scope of practice" [25, 27]. Clinical nurse specialists are registered nurses (RN) with a master's or doctoral degree in nursing, extensive nursing knowledge and skills, clinical expertise and experience in a specialty area [26, 31]. Canadian researchers report that Canada is not fully optimizing CNSs and NPs expertise in healthcare, including cancer control [17]

Nurses in Canada are regulated at the provincial or territorial level. Specific titles used in reference to ANP roles vary among provinces and territories. Currently, the only advanced practice nursing role with additional regulation and title protection, beyond RN, is the NP. Nurse practitioner legislation currently exists in all provinces and territories in Canada and national core competencies for the nurse practitioner role were revised in 2010 [28]. The number of licensed NPs in Canada has grown by more than 300 % over the past 10 years from 976 in 2006 to 4353 in 2015, with a 94 % employment rate [22]. According to a national survey, nearly three in five Canadians had a medium level of confidence and more than one in four had a high level of confidence in the ability of nurse practitioners to manage their day-to-day needs outside of hospitals [92].

There has been significant progress on a number of the recommendations and overall evolution of the NP role since the Canadian Nurse Practitioner Initiative (CNPI) [32]. NPs are now deployed across a wide variety of settings, sectors, and in various models of care. This is supported by significant harmonization and expansion of the scope of practice across jurisdictions as well as pan-Canadian title protection, a common role description, and adequate professional liability coverage – all recommended by CNPI. Among the remaining challenges to NP integration, continued advocacy is needed on federal legislative or policy barriers, e.g.: distribution of medicine samples, medical forms for disability claims and workers' compensation [32]. The number of NP education programs over the last 10 years has grown with 28 NP programs as of 2013-2014 [20]. Stakeholders view standardization of master's education as a significant success in the advancement of the NP role in Canada. As recommended by CNPI [23, 25], Canada now has national NP workforce and education data.

The clinical nurse specialist role in Canada was introduced to respond to increased patient need, a demand for nursing specialization and to support nursing practice at the point of care. CNSs provide support for quality practice and health system strengthening across the healthcare continuum. However, despite the fact that it has been part of the Canadian healthcare system for the past four decades [42], clinical nurse specialists continue to face challenges [76]. It is difficult to report the numbers for the clinical nurse specialist in Canada since the CNS title is not protected [76]. In 2014, 514 self-reported CNSs were prepared at the graduate level [22]. Results of a National Survey on CNSs in Canada identify strategies to accurately track CNSs and achieve greater consensus on a CNS role definition and educational preparation across the country [76]. Researchers in Canada also report concerns with CNSs not being fully utilized in our healthcare system.

The challenge reported by CNSs is that their work varies in each healthcare jurisdiction and the title "clinical nurse specialist" is not used consistently. The Canadian Nurses Association led the development of the first Core Competencies for the clinical nurse specialist in Canada [31]. Roundtable discussion identified that the varied use of the clinical nurse specialist role stems from confusion about what it entails. Yet, there is significant evidence demonstrating the positive contributions that clinical nurse specialists make to the health of Canadians [21]

Canadians need high quality care—care that is timely, client-centered, evidence-informed, and accessible. Better care is achievable by optimizing the roles of nurse practitioners and clinical nurse specialist in primary, community, long-term, and acute care [28, 29]. Access to care is best met by knowledgeable and skilled clinicians who can respond appropriately to complex population and individual needs. Although there continues to be a lack of understanding among healthcare professionals and the public in relationship to ANP, the professional and policy environment in Canada is generally receptive and looking to integrate a variety of ANP roles into the healthcare system. Policymakers, decision makers, and nursing are working together to face future challenges as they refine and coordinate what this means in terms of services for the country. Despite such progress there remains some limitations, nevertheless there is an opportunity to continue to advance the role to improve access to care for the health and wellbeing of Canadians in a cost effective manner. (J. Roussel, Senior Nurse Advisor, Canadian Nurses Association, 27 May 2016, personal communication)

2.4.3 Advanced Nursing Practice in Israel

Israel is a small country situated in the heart of the Middle East, consisting of approximately eight million people [35]. The government of the State of Israel is a parliamentary democracy with a healthcare system based on socialized medicine. Each resident is entitled to a basic "basket" of healthcare services from pre-cradle to grave. Services include in-patient and out-patient care, treatments, testing, and medications. Not all treatments and services are included in the "basket"; therefore many citizens pay out of pocket for private supplementary healthcare insurance and services. Community based healthcare services are provided by four Health Funds; and in-patient services by government, private, and Health Fund-owned hospitals.

Nurses serve as the largest sector of healthcare providers, similar to many westernized healthcare systems [27]. However, there is no Israeli Nurse Practice Act. All nurses practice under a clause of the Physician Practice Act passed during the establishment of the state in 1947 and revised in 1976. Therefore, the scope of nursing practice is not specifically defined by law but by executive order of the Ministry of Health and by institutional policies. The Division of Nursing within the Ministry of Health registers nurses who have successfully completed a course of study and have passed a qualifying exam. There are registries for licensed practical nurses, registered nurses, post-basic nursing certification, and advanced practice nurses [87]. Over 30 years ago the Ministry of Health initiated a policy to phase out all licensed practical nurses and require all registered nurses to obtain a baccalaureate degree. This policy has advanced nursing practice greatly; however, recently the policy has been diverted due to a severe nursing shortage. According to the Organization for Economic Cooperation and Development (OECD), there is a ratio of 4.9 nurses per 1000 population, way below the 9.1 OECD average [100].

Despite the severe shortage of nurses, the level of healthcare in Israel is considered on par with many western countries, as evidenced by Israel's life expectancy statistics that are higher than the OECD mean (80.3 for men and 81.9 for women, OECD, 2015) [100]. Such a system requires nurses to practice at a high technical and professional level. In order to produce such nurses in an environment of nursing shortages, the Ministry of Health created a system of post-basic certification. Registered nurses with some clinical experience and a baccalaureate degree can complete a post-basic certification program (usually meeting twice weekly for about 1 year, that includes both clinical and theoretical content). The content of the program is determined by the Ministry of Health and is not within an academic framework. Certifications in midwifery, operating room, intensive care, and dialysis are required of nurses who wish to work in these clinical areas while other areas such as geriatrics and oncology are voluntary.

The introduction of advanced practice came late to Israel. In 2009 an executive order was published allowing for the role of Nurse Specialist in Palliative Care [85]. Requirements for the role are a baccalaureate and master's degree (where at least one degree is in Nursing), post-basic certification in Oncology or Geriatrics, an advanced palliative care course and successful completion of a theoretical and clinical exam. Initially a group of 35 nurses who were known to practice palliative care and had post-basic certification were grandfathered in as specialists. Since that time, a few palliative courses have been given and at present there are 59 registered Palliative Care Nurse Specialists [88].

In 2011, the second role, that of Geriatric Nurse Specialist was added. At present only one geriatric specialist course was completed with 19 nurses currently registered as Geriatric Nurse Specialists. In 2013, the Ministry of Health published an executive order standardizing the specialist role within the healthcare system [86]. This document not only lists the requirements for the role but also states its scope of practice. Specialists are allowed to stop and maintain existing drug regimens, prescribe new medications for hospitalized patients, provide standard care (including admissions, follow-up care and preparation for discharge), order medical tests and blood work, request consultations from other specialties, and refer patients to the emergency room. The specialist reports professionally to the medical director of the unit but administratively falls within the purview of nursing. Specialists cannot independently discharge a patient from the hospital, start new medications in the community, nor may they sign a death certificate [86]. Since 2013, several other specialist roles have been developed, including diabetes ($n = 16$ specialists), neonatology ($n = 16$) and surgery ($n = 17$) [88]. Other specialties that are in the planning phases are rehabilitation, internal medicine, pain, primary care, and administration and policy [88].

Several factors related to the implementation of advanced practice should be noted. Firstly, before the official introduction of the specialist role into the healthcare system, many nurses performed several if not all aspects of the role. For example, wound care nurses diagnosed and treated most aspects of wound care without direct medical supervision. Secondly, while the scope of practice for the nurse specialist has been widened substantially from that of the registered nurse with postbasic certification, many nurse specialists continue to practice nursing in a staff nurse role and are not implementing the full extent of their expanded scope of practice, often due to constraints and barriers in their work environment. Thirdly, training for the advanced practice role is not within an academic framework. In other words, a nurse specialist might have a master's degree in public health or nursing administration and is not required to have a degree in advanced practice nursing. This last fact is unusual in that most countries require a master's degree in advanced practice for licensure at this level. As of June 2016, a clinical master's program has existed for 15 years but has not received the Ministry of Health's approval for teaching the content required for the specialist role. A new master's program for Geriatric Nurse Specialists that has been approved by the Ministry of Health is undergoing approval by the Higher Education Commission, a requirement for all new academic programs, and is expected to open in the 2016-7 academic year.

In summary, despite severe nursing shortages and a late start, the introduction and development of the advanced practice role in Israel is moving at a rapid pace. It is hoped that the role continues to develop, that it becomes incorporated into an academic framework, and that increased numbers of nurses are willing and authorized to perform the role. (F. DeKeyser Ganz, Coordinator, Research and Development, Hadassah-Hebrew University School of Nursing, Faculty of Medicine, Jerusalem, 04 May 2016, personal communication)

2.4.4 Japan: Advanced Nursing Practice Development

In Japan, there are four licenses in the nursing profession. Three of the licenses are issued by the government (the Minister of Health, Labour and Welfare): Public Health Nurse, Midwife, and Nurse. The other is the licensed practice nurse (formally called "Assistant Nurse") that is issued by the prefectural governor.

Public Health Nurses (PHNs) and midwives could be historically considered as APNs in Japan, because they require the relevant license in addition to the basic nurse license. Nurses need to receive additional education and pass the national examination for the PHN or Midwife, but work experience as a nurse is not required to be a PHN or Midwife. With the development of BSN (bachelor of science in nursing) study programs at the entry level of nursing education, PHN and Midwife have been less recognized as an APN, because it is now possible to take the licensure exams for all the three roles (Nurse, PHN, and Midwife) at the completion of the 4-year BSN program. Very recently, the education for PHNs and midwives has been shifting to master's level. However, PHN and midwife are no longer discussed in the context of APNs.

What are APNs in Japan? There is no official definition, but most nurses recognize Certified Nurse Specialists (CNSs) and Certified Nurses (CNs) as APNs. To become a CNS requires at least 5 years nursing work experience, completion of the master's program for CNSs accredited by the JANPU (Japan Association of Nursing Programs in Universities) and passing the qualifying exam run by the JNA (Japanese Nursing Association). To become a CN a nurse must have at least 5 years nursing work experience, the completion of about 6-months education program for CNs accredited by the JNA, and passing the qualifying exam run by the JNA.

The introduction of CNSs was part of the political activities within the nursing arena, that is, an initiative of a pillar of nursing scholars who studied abroad, particularly in the U.S.A. The introduction of CNSs should have a similar background to CNs but aim at improving the social status of nurses. There was no social or healthcare demand. Therefore, CNSs and CNs are not opposed by the other medical and healthcare professions, but also their influence on healthcare has been weak. The number of CNSs has not increased as many had expected. The certifying system of CNSs was initiated in 1996 and approximately 1500 (0.1 % of nurses) have CNS certification as of 2015.

Around 2006, a few nurses and surgeons in Japan started to study nurse practitioners in the U.S.A. in order to develop "team medicine," which was an idea of breaking traditional medical paternalism and enlarging nurse's scope of practice. Also, there is uneven distribution of physicians, mainly shortage of physicians in rural areas. Representative nurses and surgeons approached the government and a trial project for NP education in master's program was launched in 2008 at Oita University of Nursing and Health Sciences [53]. The number of master's programs for NP training increased to seven by 2013.

In the meantime, the movement members of the profession took various actions to amend the Act on Public Health Nurses, Midwives, and Nurses to initiate NPs legally. They faced opposition from all sides including nursing. Nurses who had contributed to development of CNSs particularly opposed the move to NPs. Their argument was that the movement members included physicians and they were afraid of development of Physician Assistants. The nursing opponents softened their attitude as the enlargement of nurse's scope of practice had become difficult and they had learned more about what NPs were.

Eventually, as of May 2016, there is no such a professional named nurse practitioner in Japan, even though the Japanese Organization of Nurse Practitioner Faculties (JONPF) provides the certifying exam for the graduates from the 7 NP programs. Instead, the Act on Public Health Nurses, Midwives, and Nurses was partially amended in October 2015, and the education system for nurses pertaining to specified medical interventions started. The specified medical interventions are limited to 38 interventions in 21 categories. The education program is not necessarily master's level and even a hospital can have a program for one category. The whole idea of the education system is procedure-oriented which, in the opinion of this resource, should not be based on education but on-the-job-training. The 7 master's NP programs adopted all the 38 interventions in 21 categories. The faculty members hope that the amendment would be the first step to the official introduction of NPs. The JANPU, which used to be the strongest nursing opponent to NPs, started to accredit master's NP program in 2016. The activities of the graduates from the 7 NP programs depend on the physician in the institution where the graduates work. Publications (mostly in Japanese) have described positive examples of NP work [53, 99] but the whole picture and future of the NP is still unclear. (M. Suzuki, Vice Director of Nursing, Cancer Institute Hospital of Japanese Foundation for Cancer Research, 08 May 2016, personal communication)

2.4.5 Latin America: International Collaboration and the State of Advanced Practice Nursing

In 2013, members of the Pan American Health Organization (PAHO), the Americas' regional office of the World Health Organization, passed Resolution CD52.R13 Human Resources for Health: Increasing Access to Qualified Health Workers In Primary Healthcare-Based Health System, urging further training and implementation of advanced practice nurses as a key strategy for Primary Healthcare system development [103]. The holistic, patient-centered model of nursing, together with an expanded scope of practice is considered to be necessary in addressing the many needs of the population regarding prevention, treatment, and palliative care.

In North America, the APN role has existed for over four decades, whereas in Latin America and the Caribbean, most nurses are trained to a baccalaureate level, as licensed or registered nurses. Many of these countries have academic master's degrees in nursing available to train nurses in research or education [96]. In 2014, another PAHO resolution, CD53/5, Rev. 2 Strategy for Universal Access to Health and Universal Health Coverage, was approved [104], outlining key strategies for improving Universal Health, including the expansion of health services. It reaffirmed the need for increased high quality, and more comprehensive human resources for health, capable of meeting the unique contextual needs of each country and its population. Since then, nursing organizations, leaders in nursing education, and some health ministries from across the Region of the Americas have shown increasing interest in moving forward with implementation of the APN role.

In order to move this agenda forward, the Universal Access to Health and Universal Health Coverage: Advanced Practice Nursing Summit was hosted in 2015 by PAHO/WHO and the Collaborating Center in Primary Healthcare & Health Human Resources at McMaster University in Hamilton, Canada. At this summit, participants from across the region representing health ministries, nursing associations, and nursing schools highlighted the contributions of nursing, with specific focus on APN implementation and roles in different countries, and outlined priorities for APN implementation [105]. The planning priorities for this summit included, "establishing master's level APN education programs, and establishing a Pan American collaborative network to develop and implement the APN role, define and optimize complementary RN and APN roles in new models of primary healthcare, and engage and influence decision makers, legislators, and other key stakeholders" [105, p. 9]. A draft plan was created for each priority with 1 year (April 2016) and 3 year (April 2018) steps towards implementation identified.

These planning priorities were designated to guide and unify advanced practice nursing implementation efforts in the region [105]. One result was the creation of a six-part webinar series in April 2016 titled "Advanced Practice Nursing: PAHO Activities and Strategy for Development in Latin America" [106]. The Webinar was an international collaboration of PAHO with McMaster University and was simultaneously presented in English and Spanish with the goal of increasing interest and awareness of the APN role for nurses and key shareholders in Latin America [104]. Over 300 individuals registered for the series representing nursing in over 20 countries in the PAHO region.

Additionally, the 2015 summit helped to foster greater collaboration between nursing leaders and institutions in North America with those in Latin America and the Caribbean. In February 2016, the Faculty of Nursing at Pontifica Universidad Javeriana, Colombia, hosted a celebration of its 75 year anniversary titled "Posibilidades y Realidades de la Práctica Avanzada en Enfermería en Colombia Frente a la Cobertura Universal en Salud" (Possibilities and Realities of Advanced Practice Nursing in Colombia in the Face of Universal Health Coverage) in Bogota, Colombia. A PAHO representative participated in the event as a speaker and met with several leaders of nursing and the Ministry of Health to discuss the aspects that favor advanced practice nursing in Colombia in the face of universal health coverage [51].

Meanwhile in Chile, the University of the Andes has launched a master's degree Nurse Practitioner in Adult Acute Care program. While the program is focused on the APN role in tertiary care, rather than primary care, it is a historical step as the first program in Latin America that will produce graduates in line with the ICN definition of an advanced practice nurse. The program and its curriculum are a result of collaboration with Johns Hopkins Hospital and School of Nursing, Baltimore, Maryland, United States. In addition to 460 clinical hours at their home university, the students will have the opportunity to participate in an international two-week internship at Johns Hopkins Hospital, shadowing a nurse practitioner or nurse specialist to further understand their role and observe their practice [83].

Brazil has also taken the first step towards bringing in advanced practice nursing to achieve Universal Health Coverage. In November 2015, representatives from the Federal Council of Nursing and the Brazilian Nursing Association came to PAHO headquarters in Washington DC to discuss and plan the future of APN in Brazil. At this meeting, they decided to join together and write a document about the scope of the APN role in Brazil in primary healthcare to be presented to the Minister of Health. They will also organize an international seminar in June 2016 with all the nursing organizations in the country to increase visibility of the discussion in Brazil.

To follow-up on the work of the 2015 summit, PAHO/WHO and the Collaborating Center in Nursing and Midwifery at the University of Michigan School of Nursing in Ann Arbor, USA hosted "Developing Advanced Practice Nursing Competencies in Latin America to contribute to Universal Health", a 2½ day meeting in April of 2016. This meeting was built on the priorities set in 2015 by addressing APN competencies and curriculum development.

Many challenges still exist for APN implementation in Latin American and Caribbean countries. Some of these include lack of recognition of the significant role nursing has in strengthening health systems, the development of postgraduate nursing education where countries may not have existing graduate nursing courses to build from, and bringing in health reform and changes to health system policy that enable APNs to practice to their full scope of practice. That said, four decades of experience with APN implementation in Canada and the United States and other countries globally can provide crucial insight into the development of strong policies to lead to effective APN implementation in Latin America and the Caribbean. (S. Cassiani, Regional Advisor on Nursing and Allied Health Personnel, PAHO/WHO, Washington DC; L.K. Rosales, 2016 Intern Department of Health Systems and Services, PAHO/WHO Washington DC, D. Oldenburger, Research Intern, Global Health, McMaster University, Hamilton, Ontario, Canada; J. Pulcini, Director of Community and Global Initiatives, George Washington University School of Nursing, Washington DC, 28 March 2016, personal communication)

2.4.6   Oman: Development of the Advanced Practice Role

In Oman, the driving forces for advanced nursing practice include a shortfall in physicians especially in the primary healthcare (PHC) setting both in numbers and specific expertise. In addition, emerging health problems due to lifestyle changes, increase in life expectancy, and the global trend of moving care closer and deeper into the community caught the attention of the Ministry of Health. Interest in the development of the APN role was initiated in 2004. One of the strategic directives for primary healthcare (PHC) in Oman was to expand the role of nurses in care delivery by developing advanced nursing practice (ANP). The rationale for developing the role was articulated by a WHO (World Health Organization) consultant in reviewing the PHC delivery system in Oman. This was followed by a situation analysis of the role with reference to PHC by another WHO consultant in 2005 to advise nationals on the preparation for this role. The observations of both of the consultants demonstrated high utilization and heavy patient load for physicians in larger health centers that created a bottle neck of PHC services around the physician that could lead to poor outcomes and patient-provider dissatisfaction. In small health centers, however, nurses function in an extended scope of practise including minor diagnosis and treatment. Thus, when there is no physician in the health center nurses are compelled by the demand of care to prescribe and manage under the sunset rule.

In 2006, a WHO consultant with expertise in ANP visited Oman to specifically assess the potential for implementation of the role in relation to provision of healthcare services in the community. The consultant concluded that progressing to community nurse practitioner roles had the potential for strengthening community care in Oman. However, it was identified that the current nursing education does not offer preparation for those nurses who are already functioning in advanced clinical capacity. The WHO consultant revisited Oman in 2007 to review the educational system and highlight key points to consider for the future nursing workforce and educational plan. This was followed by a proposal by the WHO Eastern Mediterranean Region in 2008 to develop the role at primary, secondary, and tertiary levels of care.

In 2010, the Directorate General of Nursing Affairs built on the previous work of the WHO consultants took a triangulated approach in order to gather evidence and support the development of the ANP role. The first phase was a situational analysis of the extended role of the PHC nurses. Information in terms of specific advanced practice skills was gathered and analyzed.

The process of gathering information was supplemented by the second phase, a focus group discussion in 2011 involving key stake holders from service, education, and professional regulation in order to come to a consensus regarding the need of the population, optimal educational preparation, career path and progression and regulation of practice nationally. The discussions were supplemented by a review on relevant international literature. A consultation process with decision makers and key stake holders at the Ministry of Health took place in October 2011. The recommendations of this consultation was to widen the scope of needs assessment in order to identify expected competencies, scope of practice, career pathway, professional role, and number of nurse practitioners required nationally.

This led to the third phase in December 2011 of studying the perceptions of the healthcare professionals with regards to the ANP role. The population for the study included physicians, nurses, lab technicians, and pharmacists working in PHC, educators from the Directorate of Education and Training (DGET), Regulators from the Oman Nursing and Midwifery Council (ONMC), stakeholders, and Program Directors from the Ministry of Health Headquarters. The results of the study demonstrated that other healthcare professions are supportive of the introduction of ANP.

These three phases led to the next follow up visit by two WHO consultants in April 2012. The aim of the visit was to review and analyse documents and reports related to ANP and to meet and discuss with decision makers, educators, and practice nurses. The recommendations of the visit were twofold:

- Education of nurses functioning in the extended capacity currently prescribing and case managing in remote PHC setting
- Developing the ANP role

Exploratory discussions indicated that the current situation in Oman would require considerable strengthening and support to implement the program and thus initially it was agreed that outside consultation would be necessary. Two models of practice were introduced:

- Model 1: Depicts a trajectory that the registered nurse could follow from the extended through the specialist to the ANP role
- Model 2: Depicts the targets of care and the levels for referral for the family health nurse practitioner

As per the recommendations of the consultants, a multidisciplinary taskforce was created to establish an agreement on the key areas of role development and to monitor and evaluate the progress of ANP in PHC initially and in secondary and tertiary level at a later date. However, the decision-makers and the stakeholders at the Ministry of Health suggested studying the need for the role in the hospital setting first. The Directorate General of Nursing Affairs carried out an in-depth literature review in this regard. Based on the evidence gathered it was strongly believed that there is an emerging need to develop this role in the PHC setting initially and then in the hospital setting at a later stage. The taskforce came to a consensus to identify and empower nurses legally to practice within boundaries of a well-defined scope of practice. Criteria for selection and preparation of these nurses were discussed. A mapping activity was performed to identify nurses currently engaged in extended role practices with a decision to train them on the job.

Following the 2012 consultancy visit, the proposal of introducing the ANP role and integrating it in the healthcare workforce plan was submitted to the decision makers for approval and feedback. Based on their positive response, a follow-up visit by the WHO consultant was scheduled to guide the development of a training program for nurses practicing in the extended role and in developing the ANP role including the scope and standards of practice, service delivery structure, practice environment, and legal framework in March 2016. (M. Al-Maqbali, Directorate General of Nursing Affairs, Ministry of Health Oman, 07 April 2016, personal communication)

2.4.7   South Africa: Advanced Psychiatric Nursing, a New Specialty

An identified rationale for an advanced nurse practitioner role in South Africa stimulated interest in advanced psychiatric nursing. It is estimated that one in every three South Africans are suffering from some form of mental illness. There is a lack of mental health professionals in the public and private healthcare domain to treat these individuals [147]. In assessing the need for this new nursing role, attention was paid to multiple studies and meta-analysis reviews that concluded care provided by advanced practice nurses is comparable or equivalent in quality to the care provided by physicians [94, 135]. It is anticipated that training a specialist psychiatric nurse practitioner with expert and advanced knowledge and clinical skills will promote the health status of the South African population and alleviate the lack of skills and practitioners in order to address the burden in the healthcare system.

The focus of education is on adult psychiatry and incorporates two electives – child and adolescent as well as forensic psychiatric nursing. The curriculum draws on various developmental and nursing theories designed to prepare graduates in advanced physiology/pathophysiology, psychopharmacology, mental health assessment, diagnosis of mental health conditions, case management, crisis intervention, milieu and psychotherapy (e.g., counseling/debriefing, individual, group, family couple, and cognitive behavior), psychosocial rehabilitation, consultation, psychoeducation, promotion of best possible mental health and prevention of mental disorders, such as assessment of risk factors for mental illness of individuals, groups, families, school learners, nursing research projects, interdisciplinary collaboration across a wide range of healthcare settings, and ethos and professional leadership.

Additionally, the practical component provides enough opportunities for intensive advanced clinical exposure in different accredited clinical facilities. As stipulated in the Psychiatric Mental Health Nursing, Scope and Standards Draft Revision [107], the practical component of the course is designed to enable students to synthesize and integrate concepts from their basic psychiatric nurse education with their advanced psychiatric knowledge foundation.

2.4.7.1 Role Qualifications

Nurses and midwives in South Africa are educated to function at both entry level and higher level in specific fields of practice. Existing nursing education provides for diplomas and advanced diplomas (additional qualifications) that culminate in professional registration with the Nursing Council. For the purpose of professional registration, the Council currently does not distinguish between a nurse who obtained the qualification through an advanced diploma qualification and the one who obtained it from a master's degree. Registration of an additional qualification for a professional nurse is currently dependent on the focus of the additional/specialized discipline, regardless of whether this was obtained through a diploma, a bachelor's degree, master's degree, or any other qualification. This has resulted in uncertainty about the status and classification of advanced practice nurses in South Africa and has implications which impact on remuneration and clinical career-paths of the advanced practice nurse [130–132].

On successful completion of this qualification, registered advanced psychiatric nurses are able to work in a variety of private as well as state domains, such as general facilities, psychiatric in-outpatient facilities, as well as in community mental healthcare centers. In addition, they can work as therapists, consultants, and case managers to render comprehensive care and treatment services to adults, children and adolescents, and families with acute/chronic psychiatric disorders, e.g., post-traumatic stress, depression, anxiety, bipolar disorder, schizophrenia and substance/alcohol abuse, neurocognitive disorders, loss/grief adjustment problems, difficulties to cope with trauma, e.g., sexual assault, gender based/domestic violence, and child and elderly abuse.

2.4.7.2 Challenges for Advanced Psychiatric Registered Nurses in the South African Context

As early as 1996 Moller and Haber [89] suggested that to move psychiatric-mental health nursing as a specialty forward, a blended advanced practice role is the most suitable because it retains the excellence of the psychosocial tradition and incorporates the biological perspective of the future. Although the curriculum for advanced psychiatric nurses in South Africa is developed as such, when these nurses return to their work places, they experience major resistance within the multidisciplinary team who continue to question their role and do not accept registered advanced psychiatric nurses as equal partners (personal communication with advanced registered nurses at different institutions in South Africa between 2011 and 2015). Some team members did not understand the difference between the scope of nursing of a basic psychiatric registered nurse and those of an advanced psychiatric registered nurse.

Findings of a South African study conducted by Doodhnath [45] revealed similar patterns. The participants in this study stated that advanced psychiatric registered nurses after completion of study were frustrated due to the demands of the regular nursing duties, specific ward demands, lack of human resources, dual responsibility, role conflict, confusion, work overload, unchanged roles/duties, increased personal and/or organizational expectations, and organizational/structural barriers which delay the implementation and practice of advanced psychiatric nurse. With lack of support from management and team members, there are limited opportunities to practice in their advanced role in South Africa.

Currently, advanced psychiatric nurses do not have prescriptive authority and they are not expected to be competent in physical assessment. However, many take additional courses to develop competence in advanced physical assessment and prescribing courses.

The role of the advanced psychiatric nurse in South Africa needs clarity and parity [101]. Therefore, to adequately act in the best interest of the public, advanced psychiatric registered nurses in South-Africa whether it is in private or in state facilities should be optimally utilized; multidisciplinary team members and nursing managers need to have a mindset change by accepting the pivotal role advanced practice psychiatric nurses can contribute to effectively address the bio psychosocial population needs in the future healthcare system of South Africa. (E. van Wijk, Western Cape College, Republic of South Africa, 17 January 2016, personal communication)

Conclusion

This chapter presents a comprehensive and detailed representation of the growing international presence of advanced nursing practice. It is not the intent of the author to reveal every circumstance of advanced nursing practice development globally; however, the extent of this trend in the provision of healthcare services is exemplified in the diversity of the country profiles. The focus of this chapter is to provide a snapshot of development and progression of advanced nursing practice to stimulate discussion and further inquiry. As the world grapples with healthcare reform and change in provision of healthcare services, aspects of this nursing phenomenon call for a universal language relevant to the discipline to aid dialogue. This chapter reveals the individual nature of initiatives in the field along with the similarities and disparities relevant to development.

References

1. Affara FA, Schober M (2012) Report on the development of the advanced practice nursing role in the Sultanate of Oman. WHO-EMRO, Cairo
2. Aiken LH, Sloane DM, Bruyneel L, Van den Heede K, Griffiths P, Busse R, DiomidousM, Kinnunen J, Kózka M, Lesaffre E, McHugh M, Moreno-Casbas MT, Rafferty AM, Schwendimann R, Scott PA, Tishelman C, van Achterberg T, Sermeus W; for the RN4CAST consortium (2014) Nurse staffing and education and hospital mortality in nine European countries: a retrospective observational study. Lancet 383(9931):1824–1830. doi:10.1016/S0140-6736(13)62631-8
3. American Association of Colleges of Nursing (AACN) (1996) The essentials of master's education for advanced practice nursing. Accessed 04 May 2016 from http://www.aacn.nche.edu/publications/order-form/masters-essentials
4. American Association of Colleges of Nursing (AACN) (2011) The Essentials of Master's Education in Nursing. Author: AACN, Washington, D.C.
5. American Association of Nurse Practitioners (AANP) (2015) NP fact sheet. Accessed 14 Mar 2016 from https://www.aanp.org/all-about-nps/np-fact-sheet
6. An Bord Altranais (2008) http://www.nmbi.ie/ECommerceSite/media/NMBI/ABA_Annual_Report_2008.pdf
7. Ang BC (2002) The quest for nursing excellence. Singapore Med J 43(10):493
8. BAG Bundesamt für Gesundheit (BAG) (2013) Gesundheit 2020 – Die gesundheitspolitischen Prioritäten des Bundesrates. Bern
9. Begley C, Murphy K, Higgins A, Elliot N, Lalor J, Sheerin F, Coyne I, Comiskey C, Normand C, Casey C, Dowling M, Devane D, Cooney A, Farrelly F, Brennan M, Meskell P, MacNella P (2010) Evaluation of clinical nurse and midwife specialist and advanced nurse and midwife practitioner roles in Ireland (SCAPE) final report. National Council for the Professional Development of Nursing and Midwifery in Ireland, Dublin
10. Berland Y (2003) Rapport "Coopération des professions de santé: le transfert de tâches et de compétences". Observatoire national de la démographie des professions de santé
11. BFH – Bern University of Applied Sciences, Master of Science in Nursing (2015). Accessed 23 Mar 2016 from www.gesundheit.bfh.ch/de/master/pflege.html
12. Boeckler U (2014) Die Zukunft von Pflege heute gestalten. Arbeitsfeld Pflegeentwicklung – auf dem Weg zu einer wirksamen Pflegepraxis. Die Diakonieschwester 1:3–8
13. Boeckler U, Dorgerloh S (2014) Advanced nursing practice: Eine Option für deutsche Kliniken. CNE Pflegemanagement 2:14–15
14. Bögli J (2014) Neue Wege gehen mit dem MSc Pflege: Christine Wyss: jeden Tag aufs Neue herausgefordert. Krankenpflege Soins Infirm 107(1):15
15. Borgès Da Silva G (2015) Maladies chroniques: vers un change- ment du paradigme des soins. Sante Publique 7(suppl 1):S9–S1
16. Bryant-Lukosius D (2016) Synthèse de politique du CII, la pratique infirmière avancée, une composante essentielle des ressources humaines nationales pour la santé. ICN
17. Bryant-Lukosius D, Cosby R, Bakker D, Earle C, Fitzgerald B, Burkoski V (2015) Effective use of advanced practice nurses in the delivery of Adult Cancer Services in Ontario. Cancer Care Ontario. Program in evidence-based care guidelines, Evidence-Based Series No. 16–4
18. Bryant-Lukosius D, Spichinger E, Martin J, Stoll H, Kellerhals SD, Fleidner M, Grossman F, Henry M, Hermann L, Koller A, Schwendimann R, Ulrich A, Weibel L, Callen SB, De Gesst S (2016) Framework for evaluating the impact of advanced practice nursing roles. J Nurs Scholarsh 48(2):201–209. doi:10.1111/jnu.12199

19. Buchan J, Temido M, Fronteira I, Lapao L, Dussault G (2013) Nurses in advanced roles: a review of acceptability in Portugal. Rev Latino-Am. Enfermagem 21(Spec):38–46

20. Canadian Association of Schools in Nursing (2015) Registered nurses education in Canada statistics 2013-2014. Author, Ottawa, Accessed from: http://www.casn.ca/wp-content/uploads/2015/11/2013-2014-SFS-draft-report-FINAL-public-copy.pdf

21. Canadian Centre for Advanced Practice Nursing Research (CCAPNR) (2012) The clinical nurse specialist: getting a good return on healthcare investment [Briefing note]. Accessed from http://fhs.mcmaster.ca/ccapnr/documents/onp_project/CNS_Brief_final.pdf

22. Canadian Institute for Health Information (2016) Regulated nurses, 2015. Author, Ottawa, Accessed 8 June 2016 from: https://secure.cihi.ca/free_products/Nursing_Report_2015_en.pdf

23. Canadian Nurses Association (CNA) (2006) Canadian nurse practitioner initiative: implementation and evaluation toolkit for nurse practitioners in Canada. Author, Ottawa

24. Canadian Nurses Association (CNA) (2008) Advanced nursing practice: a national framework. Author, Ottawa

25. Canadian Nurses Association (CNA) (2009a) Recommendations of the Canadian nurse practitioner initiative: progress report. Author, Ottawa

26. Canadian Nurses Association (CNA) (2009b) Clinical nurse specialist [position statement]. Author, Ottawa

27. Canadian Nurses Association (CNA) (2009c) Nurse practitioner [position statement]. Author, Ottawa

28. Canadian Nurses Association (CNA) (2010) Canadian Nurse Practitioner Core Competency Framework. Author: CNA, Ottawa, ON

29. Canadian Nurses Association (CNA) (2012a) Strengthening the role of the clinical nurse specialist in Canada [Background paper]. Author, Ottawa

30. Canadian Nurses Association (CNA) (2012b) National expert commission. Author, Ottawa

31. Canadian Nurses Association (CNA) (2014) Core competencies for the clinical nurse specialist. Author, Ottawa

32. Canadian Nurses Association (CNA) (2016) The Canadian nurse practitioner initiative: a 10 year retrospective. Author, Ottawa (in press)

33. CANMEDS (2016) Accessed 17 Feb 2016 from http://www.royalcollege.ca/portal/rc/canmeds/framework

34. Carey N, Stenner K (2011) Does non-medical prescribing make a difference to patients? Nurs Times 107(26):14–16

35. Central Bureau of Statistics (2015) Annual data 2015. Accessed from http://www.cbs.gov.il/reader/shnaton/shnatone_new.htm?CYear=2015

36. Chan S, Thompson DR, Wong T (2006) Nurses as agents of quality improvement. In: Leung GM, Bacon-Shone J (eds) Hong Kong's health systems: reflections, perspectives and visions. Hong Kong University press, Hong Kong

37. Debout C (2014) La filière clinique en soins infirmiers, éléments de clarification dans le contexte français. Soins 59:26–31

38. Decker L (2011) Pflegeexperten St.Franziskus Hospital Münster. Video on YouTube. Accessed 03 May 2016 from https://www.youtube.com/watch?v=yy1lBB46d_g

39. De Geest S, Moons P, Callens B, Gut C, Lindpaintner L, Spirig R (2008) Introducing advanced practice nursing/nurse practitioners in healthcare systems: a framework for reflection and analysis. Swiss Med Wkly Eur J Med Sci 138(43–44):621–628

40. Delemaire M, LaFortune G (2010) Nurses in advanced roles: a description and evaluation of experiences in 12 developed countries. OECD Health Working Papers, No. 54, OECD Publishing. doi:10.1787/5kmbrcfms5g7-en

41. Deutscher Berufsverband für Plegeberufe, Österreichischer Gesundheits und Krankenpflegeverband (ÖGKV) & Schweizer Berufsverband (2013). Advanced Nursing Practice in Deutschland, Osterreich und der Schweiz: Eine Positionierung von DBfK, OGKV und SBK. Deutscher Berufsverband fur Pflegeberyfe; Osterreichiscer Gesundheits und Krankenpflefeverband; Schweizer Berufsverband der Plegefachfrauen und Plegefachmanner. Accessed from http://www.dbfk.de/de/veroeffentlichungen/Positionspapiere.php

42. DiCenso A (2008) Roles, research & resilience: the evolution of advanced practice nursing. Canadian Nurse 104(9):37–40

43. DiCenso A, Bryant-Lukosius D, Bourgeault I, Martin-Misener R, Donald F, Abelson J, Kaasalainen S, Kilpatrick K, Kioke S, Carter N and Harbman P (2010) Clinical nurse specialists and nurse practitioners in Canada: a decision support synthesis. Available from http://www.chsrf.ca/migrated/pdf/10-CHSRF-0362_Dicenso_EN_Final.pdf

44. Directive 2013/55/EU of the European Parliament and of the Council. http://eur-lex.europa.eu/legal-content/EN/TXT/PDF/?uri=CELEX:32013L0055&from=EN

45. Doodhnath MM (2013) Experiences of advanced psychiatric nurses on their practice in an occupational specific dispensation hospital setting. Accessible from http://etd.uwc.ac.za/.../Manesh%20Doodhnath%20Dissertation%202014%2021

46. Drennan J, Naughton C, Allen D, Hyde A, Felle P, O'Boyle K, Treacy P, Butler M (2009) Independent evaluation of the nurse and midwife prescribing initiative. University College Dublin, Dublin, https://www.hse.ie/eng/services/publications/hospitals/prescribing_initiative.pdf

47. Duckett S, Breadon P, Farmer J (2014) Unlocking skills in hospitals: better jobs, more care. Grattan Institute, Melbourne, p4

48. Ens4care http://www.ens4care.eu/

49. ENS4Care (2015) Evidence based guidelines for nursing and social care on eHealth Services. Guideline on Advance Practice Roles. http://www.ens4care.eu/wp-content/uploads/2015/12/Final-ENS4Care-Guideline-3-Advanced-Roles-pv.pdf

50. ENS4Care (2015) Evidence based guidelines for nursing and social care on eHealth Services Nurse ePrescribing. http://www.ens4care.eu/wp-content/uploads/2015/07/D5-2-Final-ENS4Care-Guideline-Nurse-ePrescribing-19-06-2015.pdf

51. Facultad de Enfermería, Revista de Investigación (2016) Programa: Celebración 75 Años de la Facultad de Enfermería y 15 Años de La Revista Imagen Y Desarrollo. Manuscript

52. FHO/FH St. Gallen (2015), University of Applied Sciences, MA study program in Nursing. Accessed 3 Mar 2016 from http://www.fhsg.ch/fhs.nsf/de/msc-pflege-auf-einen-blick

53. Fukuda H, Miyauchi S, Tonai M, Ono M, Magilvy JK, Murashima S (2014) The first nurse practitioner graduate programme in Japan. INR 61(4):487–490. doi:10.1111/inr.12126

54. GDK/BAG (2012) Schweizerische Gesundheitsdirektorenkonferenz und Bundesamt fur Gesundheit. Neue Versorgungsmodelle fur die medizinische. Grundversorgung. Bericht der Arbeitsgruppe "Neue Versorgungsmodelle fur die medizinische Grundversorgung" von GDK und BAG [New models of primary care]. Bern

55. GesBG – Gesundheitsberufegesetz (New Health Professions Act), preliminary draft concerning the federal law regulating health care professions, Bundesamt for Gesundheit BAG (Swiss Federal Office of Public Health SFOPH) and Staatssekretariat für Bildung, Forschung und Innovation SBFI (State Secretariat for Education and Research SER). Accessed 03 Mar 2016 http://www.gesbg.admin.ch/index.html?lang=de)

56. Gic REPASI (2014) État des lieux des infirmières de pratique avancée, spécialistes cliniques et cliniciennes en France. Étude descriptive transversale

57. Hamric A (2005) A definition of advanced practice nursing. In: Hamric A, Spross J, Hanson C (eds) Advanced nursing practice: an integrative approach, 3rd edn. WB Saunders, Philadelphia, pp 21–41

58. Hamric A, Spross JA, Hanson CM (eds) (2009) Advanced practice nursing: an integrative approach, 4th edn. Saunders Elsevier, St Louis

59. Health Education England (HEE) (2015) The future of primary care: creating teams for tomorrow. Report by the Primary Care Workforce Commission. Access from http://www.hee.nhs.uk

60. Hemani H (2003) History of nursing in Pakistan. National nursing text book board. Peshawar, Pakistan

61. Henart L, Berland Y, Cadet D (2011) Rapport relatif aux métiers en santé de niveau intermédiaire. Professionnels d'aujourd'hui et nouveaux métiers: des pistes pour avancer

62. Hill M, Parker J (2015) Landscaping report for the development of the Chinese Advanced Nursing Practice Program. Report to the Chair, China Medical Board China Nursing Network

63. Holmboe ES, Hawkins RE (eds) (2008) Practical guide to the evaluation of clinical competence. Mosby Elsevier, Philadelphia

64. International Council of Nurses (ICN) (2001) Update: international survey of nurse practitioner/advanced practice nursing roles. Accessed 09 Mar 2016 from https://international.aanp.org/Practice/Survey2001

65. International Council of Nurses (ICN) (2008) The scope of practice, standards and competencies of the advanced practice nurse. ICN, Geneva

66. Imhof L, Naef R, Wallhagen MI, Schwarz J, Mahrer-Imhof R (2012) Effects of an advanced practice nurse in-home health consultation program for community-dwelling persons aged 80 and older. J Am Geriatr Soc 60:2223–2231. doi:10.1111/jgs.12026

67. INS–University of Basel, Institute of Nursing Science, MA program Nursing Science (2016). Accessed 23 Mar 2016 from https://nursing.unibas.ch/studium/studium-informationen/

68. INS –University of Basel, Institute of Nursing Science, Diploma of Advanced Studies ANP plus. Accessed 23 Mar 2016 from https://nursing.unibas.ch/veranstaltungen/fort-weiterbildung-am-ins/weiterbildung-anp/anp-plus-diplom/

69. IUFRS – Université de Lausanne, Institut universitaire de formation et de recherche en soins (2015). Accessed 23 Mar 2016 from https://www.unil.ch/enseignement/home/menuinst/masters/sciences-infirmieres.html

70. Jeschke S (2010) Die Rolle von akademischen Pflegekräften in der direkten Patientenversorgung – Eine notwendige Entwicklung? Pflege 63(1):19–22

71. Kalaidos Fachhochschule Schweiz, Master of Science in Nursing (2015). Accessed 23 Mar 2016 from https://www.kalaidos-fh.ch/Departement-Gesundheit/Master-of-Science-in-Nursing

72. Kambli K, Flach D, Schwendimann R, Cignacco E (2015) Health care provision in a Swiss Urban Walk-In-Clinic. Is advanced nursing practice a solution for a new model in primary care? Int J Health Prof 2(1):64–72. doi:10.1515/ijhp-2015-0006

73. Kannusamy P (2006) A longitudinal study of advanced practice nursing in Singapore. Crit Care Nurs Clin North Am 18:545–551

74. Keeling A (2009) A brief history of advanced practice nursing in the United States. In: Hamric AB, Spross JA, Hanson CM (eds) Advanced practice nursing: an integrative approach, 4th edn. Saunders Elsevier, St. Louis

75. Ketefian S, Redman RW, Hanucharurnkul S, Masterson A, Neves EP (2001) The development of advanced practice roles: implications in the international nursing community. INR 48:152–163

76. Kilpatrick K, DiCenso A. Bryant-Lukosius D, Ritchie JA, Martin-Misner R, Carter N (2013) Practice patterns and perceived impact of clinical nurse specialist role in Canada: results of a national survey. Int J Nurs Stud 50:1524–1536

77. Künzi K, Jäggi J, Dutoit L (2013) Aktueller Stand der schweizerischen Diskussion über den Einbezug von hoch ausgebildeten nichtärztlichen Berufsleuten in der medizinischen Grundversorgung, Büro für Arbeits- und Sozialpolitische Studien (BASS). Bern

78. Latter S, Blenkinsopp A, Smith A, Chapman s, Tinelli M, Gerard K, Little P, Celino N, Granby T, Nichols P, Dorer G (2011) Evaluation of nurse and pharmacist independent prescribing. Department of Health Policy Research Programme Project 016 0108. University of Southampton. http://eprints.soton.ac.uk/184777/3/ENPIPfullreport.pdf

79. Lee D, Kai CC, Chan C, Chair SY, Chan D, Fung S, Chan E (2013) The impact on patient health and service outcomes of introducing nurse consultants: a historically controlled study. BMC Health Serv Res 13:431. doi:10.1186/1472-6963-13-431

80. Lehwaldt D (2013) Advanced practice nursing: eine qualitativ hochwertige Versorgung. Praxisbeispiel Herz-Thoraxchirurgische Pflege. PflegeLeben 02–13:14–18

81. Lehwaldt D, Keinath E, Mueller A (2016) Taking the experience abroad: Advanced nursing practice education from the UK to Germany. Poster presented at the Association of Advanced Practice Educators (AAPE) UK Annual Conference, 'The impact of Inter-Professional Advanced Practitioners on Service Design and Health and social Care on 4th March 2016 at the University of Salford

82. Lim D (2005) Developing professional nursing in Singapore: a case for change. Singapore Nurs J 32(1):34–47

83. Magíster en Práctica Avanzada de Enfermería – Mención Paciente Crítico Adulto. (N.D.). Accessed 02 Mar 2016, from http://postgrados.uandes.cl/mpae/

84. McAuliffe MS, Henry B (2002) Nurse anesthesia worldwide: practice, education and regulation. Accessed 16 Feb 2016 from http://ifna-int.org/ifna/e107_files/downloads/Practice.pdf
85. Ministry of Health (2009) Executive order, palliative care nurse specialist [in Hebrew]. Accessed from http://www.health.gov.il/hozer/ND79_09.pdf
86. Ministry of Health (2013) Executive order. Nurse specialists [in Hebrew]. Accessed from http://www.health.gov.il/hozer/ND99_2013.pdf
87. Ministry of Health, Division of Nursing (2016) Nursing activity. Accessed from www.health.gov.il/unitsOffice/nursing/activity
88. Ministry of Health, Division of Nursing (2016) Annual report, 2015 Nursing Division [in Hebrew]. Accessed from http://www.health.gov.il/hozer/ND116_2016.pdf
89. Moller DM, Haber J (1996) Advanced practice psychiatric nursing: the need for a blended role. Online J Issues Nursing. Accessible http://www.nursingworld.org/MainMenuCategories/ANAMarketplace/ANAPeriodicals/OJIN/TableofContents/Vol21997/No1Jan97/ArticlePreviousTopic/AdvancedPracticePsychiatricNursing.aspx
90. Müller M, Jaggi S, Kouriaichi C, Eggenschwiler P, Mahrer-Imhof R (2010) Scope of practice of an Advanced Practice Nurse at the Swiss Epilepsy Centre. Pflege 23(6):385–391. doi:10.1024/1012-5302/a000077
91. Müller-Staub M, Zigan N, Händler-Schuster D, Probst S, Monego R, Imhof L (2015) Being cared for and caring: living with multiple chronic diseases (Leila)-a qualitative study about APN contributions to integrated care. Pflege 28(2):79–91. doi:10.1024/1012-5302/a000410
92. Nanos (2012) National representative online survey Canadians aged 18 and over for the Canadian Nurses Association. Author, Ottawa
93. National Prescribing Centre. Prescribing competency frameworks. www.npc.nhs.uk/guidance_nmp.php
94. Newhouse RP, Stanik-Hutt J, White KM, Johantgen M, Bass EB, Zangaro G, Wilson RF, Fountain L, Steinwachs DM, Heindel L, Weiner JP (2011) Advanced practice nurse outcomes 1990-2008: a systematic review. Accessible from http://www.nursingeconomics.net/ce/2013/article3001021.pdf
95. Nicca D, Moody K, Elzi L, Spirig R (2007) Comprehensive clinical adherence interventions to enable antiretroviral therapy: a case report. J Assoc Nurses AIDS Care 18(6):44–53. doi:10.1016/j.jana.2007.03.011
96. Nigenda G, Magaña-Valladares L, Cooper K, Ruiz-Lario JA (2010) Recent developments in public health in the Americas. Int J Environ Res Public Health 201(7):729–750. doi:10.3390/ijerph7030729
97. Northern Ireland Practice and Education Council for Nursing and Midwifery (NIPEC) (2016) Advanced nursing practice framework: supporting advanced nursing practice in health and social care trusts. Belfast: Author. Accessed 14 Mar 2016 from http://www.nipec.hscni.net/Image/SitePDFS/DHSSPS%20Advanced%20Nursing%20Practice%20Framework.pdf
98. Nurse and Midwives ACT (1999) Amended by Act 15 of 2005. Accessed 10 Mar 2016 from http://statutes.agc.gov.sg
99. Ono M, Miyauchi S, Edzuki Y, Saiki K, Fukuda H, Tonai M, Magilvy JK, Murashima S (2015) Japanese nurse practitioner practice and outcomes in a nursing home. INR 62(2):275–279. doi:10.1111/inr.12158
100. Organization of Economic Cooperation and Development (OECD) (2015) Health at a glance. Indicators 2015. Accessed from http://www.oecd.org/health/health-systems/health-at-a-glance-19991312.htm
101. Paisley L (1998) Clarity and parity: understanding the roles of the advanced practice psychiatric nurse. Online J Issues Nursing 3(1). Accessible from http://www.nursingworld.org/MainMenuCategories/ANAMarketplace/ANAPeriodicals/OJIN/TableofContents/Vol31998/No1June1998/ArticlePreviousTopic/UnderstandingtheRoles.aspx
102. Pakistan Ministry of Finance (2014–2015) Pakistan economic survey 2014 – 2015. Accessed 03 May 2016 from http://www.finance.gov.pk/survey/chapters_15/11_Health.pdf
103. Pan American Health Organization (PAHO) (2013) Resolution CD52.R13. human resources for health: increasing access to qualified health workers in primary health care-based health system. Accessed from http://www.paho.org/hq/index.php?option=com_docman&task=doc_download&gid=25587&Itemid

104. Pan American Health Organization (PAHO) (2014) Strategy for universal access to health and universal health coverage. Accessed from http://www.paho.org/hq/index.php?option=com_docman&task=doc_download&gid=27312&Itemid=270&lang=en9

105. Pan American Health Organization (PAHO) (2015) Report on universal access to health and universal health coverage: advanced practice nursing summit. Manuscript

106. Pan American Health Organization (PAHO) (2016) Advanced practice nursing: PAHO activities and strategy for development in Latin America Webinar 1 presentation. Accessed from https://paho.webex.com/paho/lsr.php?RCID=9753c817faec94d98df508e30653b56c

107. Psychiatric Mental Health Nursing Scope & Standards (2006) Accessible from http://www.ispn-psych.org/docs/standards/scope-standards-draft.pdf

108. Pulcini J (2014) International development of advanced practice nursing. In: Hamric AB, Hanson CM, Tracy MF, O'Grady ET (eds) Advanced practice nursing: an integrative approach. 5th edn. Elsevier Saunders, St. Louis, pp 133–145

109. Pulcini J, Jelic M, Gul R, Loke AY (2010) An international survey on advanced practice nursing education, practice and regulation. J Nurs Scholarsh 42(1):31–39

110. Rex C, Guldener Meier A, Bischofberger I (2015) Koordinierte Versorgung zahlt sich aus. Krankenpflege Soins Infirm 108(7):14–16

111. Romain-Glassey N, Ninane F, de Puy J, Abt M, Mangin P, Morin D (2014) The emergence of forensic nursing and advanced nursing practice in Switzerland: an innovative case study consultation. J Forensic Nurs 10(3):144–152. doi:10.1097/JFN.0000000000000039

112. Roodbol P (2004) Survey carried out prior to the 3rd ICN International Nurse Practitioner/Advanced Practice Nursing Network Conference. Unpublished report, Groningen

113. Royal College of Nursing (RCN) (2012) RCN competencies: advanced nurse practitioners. An RCN guide to advanced nursing practice, advanced nurse practitioners and programme accreditation. Accessed 13 Mar 2016 from http://www.rcn.org.uk/__data/assets/pdf_file/0003/146478/003207.pdf

114. Royal College of Nursing Scotland (RCN Scotland) (2015) Nurse innovators: clinical decision-making in action. Author, Edinburgh

115. Sachverständigenrat zur Begutachtung der Entwicklung im Gesundheitswesen (SVR Gesundheit) (2007) Kooperation und Verantwortung – Voraussetzungen einer zielorientierten Gesundheitsversorgung. Accessed 03 May 2016 from http://dipbt.bundestag.de/dip21/btd/16/063/1606339.pdf

116. Sastre-Fullana P, De Pedro-Gomez JE, Bennasar-Veny M, Serrano-Gallardo P, Morales-Ascencio JM (2014) Competency frameworks for advanced practice nursing: a literature review. INR 61(4):534–542

117. SBK, Swiss ANP, VfP und IUFRS-UniL – Regulation of nursing care experts APN, summary and reasons concerning the separate regulation, key issues paper oft he SBK, Swiss ANP, Schweizerischer Verein für Pflegewissenschaft VfP (Swiss Association for Nursing Science ANS) and IUFRS-UniL (2012) (Institut universitaire de formation et de recherche en soins, Université de Lausanne)

118. Schober M (2002) Advanced practice: A global perspective. Paper presented at The 2nd ICN International Nurse Practitioner/Advanced Practice Nursing Network Conference, Adelaide

119. Schober M (2007) Report on the development of advanced community nursing/nurse practitioner roles and educational programmes in Oman, EM/NUR/392/07.07, Cairo: WHO-EMRO

120. Schober M (2007) Report on the development of a framework for advanced practice Nursing in Bahrain, EM/NUR/394/E/R/07.07, Cairo: WHO-EMRO

121. Schober M (2013) Factors Influencing the development of advanced practice nursing in Singapore, Doctoral thesis, Sheffield Hallam University, Sheffield Hallam University archives. Accessed 17 Feb 2016 from http://shura.shu.ac.uk/7799/

122. Schober M, Affara F (2006) Advanced nursing practice. Blackwell Ltd, Oxford

123. Schober M, Gerrish K, McDonnell A (2016) Development of a conceptual policy framework for advanced practice nursing: an ethnographic study. J Adv Nurs 72(6):1313–1324. doi:10.1111/jan.12915

124. Schwandt T (ed) (2014) Understanding medical education: evidence, theory and practice. Wiley Blackwell, London

125. Scottish Government (2008) Supporting the development of advanced nursing practice: a toolkit approach. Scottish Government, Author
126. Serena A, Castellani P, Fucina N, Griesser AC, Jeanmonod J, Peters S, Eicher M (2015) The role of advanced nursing in lung cancer: a framework based development. Eur J Oncol Nurs 19(6):740–746. doi:10.1016/j.ejon.2015.05.009
127. Sheer B, Wong F (2008) The development of advanced nursing practice globally. J Nurs Scholarsh 40(3):204–211
128. Shiu AT, Lee DT, Chau JP (2012) Exploring the scope of expanding advanced nursing practice in nurse-led clinics: a multiple case study. J Adv Nurs 68(8):1780–1792. doi:10.1111/j.1365-2648.2011.05868.x
129. Sibanda S (2013) ICN nurse practitioner/advanced practice nursing network country profiles. Accessed 13 Mar 2016 from http://international.aanp.org/Content/docs/CountryProfiles2014. pdf
130. South African Nursing Council (SANC). Regulations: course in clinical nursing science. Accessible from http://www.sanc.co.za/regulat/Reg-cln.htm
131. South Africa Nursing Council (SANC) (2012) Advanced practice nursing (position statement). Accessible from http://www.sanc.co.za/position_advanced_practice_nursing
132. South African Nursing Council (SANC) (2014) Competencies –generic competency framework for advanced nurse practitioners. Accessible from www.sanc.co.za/.../Competencies/ SANC%20Competencies-Generic%20F
133. Spirig R (2010) 10 Jahre Advanced Nursing Practice in der Schweiz: Rückblick und Ausblick. Pflege 23(6):363–366. doi:10.1024/1012-5302/a000075
134. Spross JA (2014) Conceptualizations of advanced practice nursing. In: Hamric AB, Hanson CM, Tracy MF, O'Grady ET (eds) Advanced practice nursing: an integrative approach, 5th edn. Elsevier, St Louis
135. Swan M, Ferguson S, Chang A, Larson E, Smaldone A (2015) Quality of primary care by advanced practice nurses: a systematic review. Accessible from http://www.intqhc.oxford-journals.org/content/early/2015/08/02/intqhc.mzv054
136. Swiss ANP – Advanced Practice Nursing, role profiles for APN nursing care experts in Switzerland. Interest group for Advanced Nursing Practice. Accessed 23 Mar 2016 from http://www.swiss-anp.ch
137. The Federal Council of Switzerland. Accessed 29 Mar 2016 from https://www.news.admin. ch/message/index.html?lang=de&msg-id=61069
138. The Swiss Parliament. Accessed 29 Mar 2016 from https://www.parlament.ch/de/services/ news/Seiten/20160302113401301194158159041_bsd108.aspx
139. Teigeler B (2015) Mit Master am Patientenbett. Die Schwester Der Pfleger 53 Jahrg.1/14
140. Ullmann P, Lehwaldt D (2013) Hochschulische Masterprogramme im Kontext der modernen Pflegebildung – die nationale Perspektive. (I Darmann-Finck, M Hülsken-Giesler, Hrsg.) Accessed 23 Apr 2016 from http://www.bwpat.de/ht2013/ft14/ullmann_lehwaldt_ft14-ht2013.pdf
141. Ullmann P, Thissen K, Ullmann B, Schwerdt R, Haynert H, Grissom B, Keogh J, Lehwaldt D, Schmitte H, Merki D, Haider AZ, Platt P, Williams D, Meier R, Holzknecht A (2011) Deutschen netzwerk advanced practice nursing & advanced nursing practice positionspapier 'Die kopernikanische Wende' advanced practice nursing, advanced nursing practice. DNAPN, Witten
142. Ullmann P, Lehwaldt D, Thissen K, Ullmann B (2013) Kongressdokumentation – 2. Internationaler Kongress Advanced Practice Nursing & Advanced Nursing Practice "Bleibt alles anders" Aufgaben und Kompetenzen von Advanced Practice Nurses im deutschsprachigen Raum. Goch: DN APN & ANP g.e.V
143. Ullmann P, Lehwaldt D, Thissen K, Ullmann B, Gantschnig G, Fierens A, Keinath E (2015) Congress Book 3rd International Congress APN, ANP, APNs – To be or not to be – activities and competencies of advanced practice nurses. DN APN & ANP g.e.V, Goch
144. Ulrich A, Hellstern P, Kressig RW, Eze G, Spirig R (2010) Advanced Nursing Practice in daily nursing care: practice development of an acute geriatric Advanced Nursing Practice team. Pflege 23(6):403–410. doi:10.1024/1012-5302/a000079

145. University of Southampton (2011) Wide-reaching report finds strong support for nurse and pharmacist prescribing http://www.southampton.ac.uk/news/2011/05/strong-support-for-nurse-and-pharmacist-prescribing.page

146. Upvall M J, Karmaliani R, Pirani F, Gul R, Khalid F (2004) Developing nursing leaders through graduate education in Pakistan. Int J Nursing Educ Scholar 1(1):Article 27. doi:10.2202/1548-923x.1079

147. Volmink H (2014) Critical shortage of mental health professionals in SA. Accessible from http://www.politicsweb.co.za/.../critical-shortage-of-mental-health-professional

148. World Health Organization (WHO) (2015) WHO progress report on nursing and midwifery 2013–2015. Author, Geneva, Accessed 16 February 2016 from http://www.who.int/hrh/nursing_midwifery/nurse_midwifery-report/en/

149. World Health Organization – Eastern Mediterranean (WHO – EMRO) (2001) Report on the fifth meeting of the regional advisory panel on nursing and consultation on advanced practice nursing and nurse prescribing: Implications for regulation, nursing education and practice in the Eastern Mediterranean Region, WHO-EM/NUR/348/E/L. Author, Cairo

150. ZHAW – Zurich University of Applied Sciences, MA study program in Nursing (MSc) (2015). Accessed 23 Mar 2016 from http://gesundheit.zhaw.ch/de/gesundheit/studium/master/pflege.html

151. Zigan N, Imhof L, Müller V, Seitz J (2012) Nursing guided patient care pathways. Patient oriented care from admission to discharge. Krankenpflege Soins Infirm 105(5):15–17

152. Zúñiga F, Jenni G, Wiesli U, Schwendimann R (2010) Development of the role of an Advanced Practice Nurse in the long-term care of elderly people in Switzerland. Pflege 23(6):375–383. doi:10.1024/1012-5302/a000076

153. Zweifel A, Stoll HR, Jermann P, Steudter E (2014) Klinisches Assessment für die Pflegepraxis – Teil 4: Verbleib in der häuslichen Umgebung ermöglichen. Krankenpflege Soins Infirm 107(5):22–25

Nature of Practice

3

Abstract

This chapter provides an overview of attributes associated with advanced nursing practice and advanced practice nursing roles. Identifying these key features provides a means to portray and explain this level of nursing and associated nursing roles to the public, other healthcare professionals, and key decision makers. The chapter begins by explaining the significance of title protection then presents role characteristics, scope of practice, and competencies for the advanced practice nurse. The implications of three controversial issues (prescriptive authority, diagnosing, hospital privileges) are discussed. The topics of advanced tasks versus critical thinking and task reallocation related to integration of APNs within a country's healthcare workforce conclude the chapter.

Keywords

Titles • Scope of practice • Competency • Prescriptive authority • Diagnosis • Critical thinking • Task reallocation

This chapter provides an overview of attributes associated with ANP and the APN roles. Identifying these features provides a means to portray and explain this nursing role to the public, other healthcare professionals and key healthcare decision makers. The chapter begins by explaining the significance of title protection then presents role characteristics, scope of practice, and competencies for the APN. The implications of three controversial issues (prescriptive authority, diagnosing, hospital privileges) are discussed. The topics of advanced tasks and task reallocation related to integration of APNs within a country's healthcare workforce concludes the chapter.

3.1   Titles

Consensus on what title to use to designate the nurse with advanced practice credentials is fundamental when launching an ANP initiative in order to reduce confusion
when introducing a new professional to the healthcare workforce. Conferring a title
designates a certain level of confidence with respect to accountability and service
that this professional can provide. A clearly identifiable and legally protected title
safeguards the public from unqualified practitioners who have neither the education
nor competencies implied by a title. This designation also provides a way to differentiate the APN from other nursing roles [59]. In emphasizing the need to use standardized language for nursing, Clark and Lang [15] wrote that "If we cannot name
it, we cannot control it, teach it, finance it or put it into public policy" (p.109). This
perspective applies to identifying a recognized and protected title for nurses working at an advanced level of practice. Once there is consensus on a title, the additional
definition, scope of practice, competencies, and professional regulation can be
developed relevant to the title.

Unfortunately, internationally there is a lack of consensus regarding one distinct
title for all nurses practicing at an advanced level. The choice of a title appears to be
country and context sensitive (Refer to Chap. 2 for country specific examples).
Worldwide, titles are often used interchangeably, and attempting to identify the
nature of practice based on title alone can be challenging and requires a need to look
at the full profile of a designated APN in any country. In a survey of 32 countries
conducted by Pulcini et al. [50], 13 different titles were listed as representing
ANP. The most commonly used titles were nurse practitioner (44 %) and APN
(17 %). Other titles named by 86 respondents included: advanced nurse practitioner,
clinical nurse specialist, nurse specialist, professional nurse, expert nurse, certified
registered nurse practitioner, chief professional nurse with post-basic training in
primary healthcare, nurse consultant, specialist nurse practitioners, primary healthcare nurse, and advanced nurse in a specialty (p. 35). Findings from this survey did
not link role characteristics to the various identified titles, thus adding to international intrigue in continuing to seek role clarity for ANP.

Having noted the differences in titling worldwide, the significance of identifying
role characteristics and a scope of practice to define APN function in the healthcare
workforce becomes eminently important. Nevertheless, a representative and legally
protected title is the quickest method to communicate to other healthcare professionals, managers, administrators, lay personnel, and the public who this healthcare
professional is [51].

Literature indicates that when little distinction is made in identifying APN roles
from other extended or specialized nursing practice roles, development tends to
proceed in an uncertain manner [20, 22, 54]. Furthermore, based on a study conducted in Canada [19] confusion about role titles and associated lack of role clarity
for APNs posed major barriers to role integration into a recognizable position in
the healthcare workforce. "Title confusion" (Donald et al. [20], p. 191) implies that
one role title may be confused with another leading to "lack of role clarity" and
poorly defined role components. A recommendation emerges that consistent use of

titles and clear role definitions could facilitate a more complete use of APNs [20, 39].

However, in Canada where clinical nurse specialist (CNS) and nurse practitioner (NP) titles and roles coexist, Donald et al. [20] found lack of support for a single title such as APN. Study respondents indicated a preference to have clear and consistent use of titles already in use to reduce confusion to coworkers and the public. One recommendation to decrease confusion is to link titles and role descriptions to healthcare goals by using a framework to guide this process. The PEPPA (participatory, evidence-based, patient-focused process for advanced practice nursing role development, implementation, and evaluation) framework proposes such guidance [8]. An overview of the PEPPA framework can be found in Chap. 5.

3.2 Role Characteristics

Role characteristics can be viewed as features that make the APN role recognizable. In referring to key characteristics of ANP Schober [53] offered the following comments:

> What characterizes advanced nursing practice is knowledge and expertise, clinical judgment, skilled and self-initiated care and scholarly inquiry, ... not [only] job descriptions, title or setting (p.3).

At the time that ICN proposed a definition for APN roles, a set of associated characteristics in the domains of education, practice, and regulation were also presented [28]. This set of characteristics is seen as a guideline to aim for noting the necessity to make a clear distinction between characteristics of advanced versus basic nursing practice. In assessing the situation in Australia and New Zealand, Gardner et al. [22] noted that APN characteristics need to be well articulated and defined in the initial phases of development. (See Chap. 1 for the ICN APN definition and role characteristics).

Nursing leaders, researchers, and educators point out that while the core of ANP is based on nursing principles and expertise, there is an overlap with skills that have been traditionally attributed to other professions [17, 22, 45, 54]. In countries such as Canada and the USA where ANP includes a presence of both clinical nurse specialists (CNS) and nurse practitioners (NP), both roles have common characteristics with medicine but the overlap appears to be more significant with the APN practicing more autonomously in primary healthcare or out of hospital settings. However, regardless of this overlap, ANP "is not the junior practice of medicine" [58]. Accepting expressions such as "physician substitutes," "mini-doctors," "maxi-nurses," "mid-level providers," or "physician extenders" focuses on those characteristics that seem similar to traits associated with medicine but in the current international context are considered to be inappropriate and misleading AANP 2015a [1]. The tendency to continually compare APN practice with medical practice can contribute to an adversarial relationship between professionals that are intended to work collaboratively.

Delamaire and LaFortune [18] suggest that research studies need to expand from comparing how advanced practice nurses do a certain set of tasks compared with physicians, to looking more broadly at the overall coordination of care linked to positive outcomes including APN sensitive indicators. The author advocates that it is the coming together of nursing values, principles, and expertise along with advanced knowledge, clinical judgment, and decision-making skills that form the essence of ANP. This merger of elements of nursing and medicine, as exhibited in ANP, contributes an added dimension and enhanced value to the provision of health-care services.

Even though the authority to carry out advanced tasks may be beneficial to provision of healthcare services, emphasis on tasks should not be considered as the fundamental feature distinguishing ANP from basic registered nurse practice. Refer to additional sections in this chapter for discussions of defining an APN scope of practice and identifying competencies. In attempting to conceptualize ANP, the use of a model or framework can be useful in depicting the nature of APN roles. The Hamric model (Fig. 3.1) and the Brown framework (Fig. 3.2) are presented as illustrations of this approach.

The current Hamric model [58] was originally based on an early model derived from the clinical nurse specialist role [25]. Changes in practice and a better understanding of a theoretical basis for ANP are reflected in the present model (see Fig. 3.1). The Hamric model proposes an integrative understanding of the core principles of advanced nursing practice emphasizing the dynamic nature of this conceptual model while demonstrating the inherent stability of ANP. This model is widely cited in the American as well as the international advanced practice literature [40, 41, 58].

Brown [7] provides a conceptual framework (See Fig. 3.2) that is comprehensive in including environments that impact practice and the context in which practice occurs. This framework explicates the relevant components by defining building blocks, articulated assumptions, and linkages among concepts. The importance of a nursing orientation is noted, especially when APNs perform activities traditionally performed by physicians. Clinical care is the focus of the framework moving from the identification of role legitimacy to the evaluation of outcomes. Brown's framework has been cited in additional international research on ANP [23].

3.3 Scope of Practice

The scope of practice for an APN depicts the range of activities related to recognized professional responsibilities that are in keeping with boundaries imposed by regulations in the context where practice occurs [55]. "By definition the term *Scope of Practice* describes practice limits and sets parameters within which nurses in the various advanced practice nursing specialties may legally practice" (Hanson [27], p. 561). In identifying a foci or specialty, the APN scope of practice can be viewed as a generalist as in the provision of services in primary healthcare and family practice with the concentration on populations across the lifespan or as an APN who specializes in a field such as oncology, critical care, or mental health. This

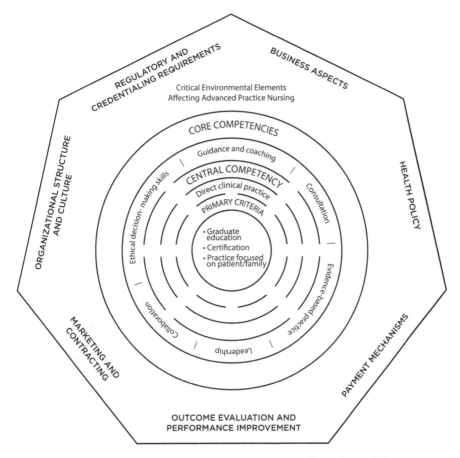

Fig. 3.1 Based on Hamric's model of advanced practice nursing (Spross [58], p 44)

distinction is commonly based on country and regional contexts, maturity of the discipline where the APN practices, population needs, and increasingly on graduate level education that is focused on knowledge and skills in a specialty.

A specialty nurse that is not defined as an APN is viewed as a registered nurse (RN) with basic nursing education plus acquired knowledge and skills to practice in a specialty. The difference between the APN in a specialty and the RN specialized is related to the depth of knowledge and critical thinking skills associated with the APN versus the RN. In an effort to promote yet differentiate the range of knowledge, skills, and competencies expected of healthcare workers, ICN developed a care continuum framework from the perspective of nursing roles [31]. In developing this framework, the ICN competencies for the generalist nurse [30] have been used as the benchmark against which other competencies for RN specialized and APN have been identified. In addition, ICN has developed a framework for the nurse specialist (RN specialized) emphasizing that qualification for these roles is greater than that acquired during basic nursing education and focused exclusively on

ENVIRONMENTS: Society, Health Care Economy, Local Conditions,
Nursing, Advanced Practice Community

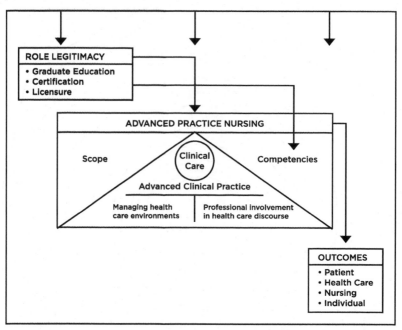

Fig. 3.2   Brown's framework for advanced practice nursing (Brown [7])

specialty practice [33]. The competencies for RN specialized were developed by
ICN for a nurse who has narrowed their focus of knowledge and skill and is working
in a distinctly specialist clinical role. Specialty expertise for this level of nursing is
obtained through a professionally approved program that leads to recognized qualifications, not usually a graduate level program.

In order to differentiate APN practice, scope of practice statements define what
APNs can do, what population can be seen or treated, and under what circumstances
the APN can provide care. Ethical and cultural contexts, educational preparation,
and accountability for professional behavior form components of the scope of practice. The scope of practice provides guidance and direction to nurses, educators,
regulatory authorities, and the public. Once defined, the scope and associated role
competencies are linked to a designated title and form the foundation for developing
suitable ANP education and the parameters of the nature of practice.

Where the ANP concept is recognized, establishment of a scope of practice is
one means of informing the public, administrators, managers, and other healthcare
professions about the role in order to differentiate the qualified APN from other
practitioners who are not adequately prepared for APN practice, or have not been
authorized to practice in this capacity. Specifying an APN scope can also assist
governments, healthcare planners, and healthcare institutions with healthcare workforce planning [32].

Scope of practice statements should communicate:

- The acquired knowledge and expertise expected of the healthcare provider
- The roles expected of the healthcare provider
- The identity of the patient population in terms of complexity of healthcare that is to be the focus and the comprehensiveness of services required
- The degree of accountability and authority that the healthcare provider assumes for practice outcomes

(Schober and Affara [55])

The Nursing Council of New Zealand provides the following illustration of a scope of practice statement for applicants who want to register as a nurse practitioner in the country:

Nurse practitioners are expert nurses who work within a specific area of practice incorporating advanced knowledge and skills. They practice both independently and in collaboration with other healthcare professionals to promote health, and prevent disease, and to diagnose, assess and manage people's health needs. They provide a wide range of assessment and treatment interventions, including differential diagnoses, ordering, conducting and interpreting diagnostic and laboratory tests, and administering therapies for the management of potential or actual health needs. They work in partnership with individuals, families, whānau and communities across a range of settings. Nurse practitioners prescribe medicines within their specific area of practice. Nurse practitioners also demonstrate leadership as consultants, educators, managers and researchers, and actively participate in professional activities, and in local and national policy development.

(NCNZ [47], p3)

Requirements for registration in New Zealand and recommended criteria that NPs must follow to identify the area and breadth of their practice follows the scope of practice the applicant provides in their application for registration document.

In proposing a professional organization's statement on scope of practice, the American Association of Nurse Practitioners AANP [2] offers a similar broad based perspective:

Nurse practitioners (NPs) are licensed independent practitioners who practice in ambulatory, acute and long-term care as primary and/or specialty care providers. Nurse practitioners assess, diagnose, treat and manage acute episodic and chronic illnesses. NPs are experts in health promotion and disease prevention. They order, conduct, supervise and interpret diagnostic and laboratory tests, prescribe pharmacological agents and non-pharmacologic therapies, as well as teach and counsel patients, among other services.

As licensed independent practitioners, nurse practitioners practice autonomously and in coordination with healthcare professionals and other individuals. They may serve as healthcare researchers, interdisciplinary consultants and patient advocates. NPs provide a wide range of healthcare services to individuals, families, groups and communities.

This scope of practice offered from this professional body adds additional aspects of education, accountability, and responsibility considered to be essential for NP practice [1, 2]. Since this scope originates from a professional association not a regulatory body it is viewed as a guideline versus a legal requirement.

The scope of practice for a Clinical Nurse Specialist (CNS) contrasts somewhat with the previous scopes of practice in that the essence of the CNS is embedded in a specialty with specialized CNS practice building on core components for all APNs plus educational experience based on a selected focus area. The CNS scope of practice is less likely to extend into the medical domain and does not usually include independent diagnosis of disease or medical conditions. The National Association of Clinical Nurse Specialists [46] in the USA provides the following scope of practice for the CNS:

> Clinical Nurse Specialists (CNSs) are registered nurses who have graduate level nursing preparation at master's or doctoral level as a CNS. CNSs are expert clinicians in a specialized area of nursing practice. The specialty may be identified in terms of: population (e.g. pediatrics, geriatrics, women's health); an identified setting (e.g. critical care, emergency room); a disease or medical subspecialty (e.g. diabetes, oncology); a type of care (e.g. psychiatric, rehabilitation) or type of problem (e.g. pain, wound, stress). The CNS practices in a wide variety of healthcare settings. In addition to providing direct patient care the CNS influences care outcomes by providing expert consultation for nursing staff and implementing improvements in healthcare delivery systems (p.2).

An APN scope of practice is built on the scope of practice defined for the generalist registered nurse and aims to distinguish how the scope of ANP expands beyond that of the registered nurse in terms of roles, functions, mastery, expertise, client populations, and accountability. Points to consider when setting out to develop an advanced scope of practice include:

- Does the scope contribute to population needs in utilization of ANP services?
- Is the scope consistent with the standards for nursing in the country and based on a core body of nursing knowledge?
- Does the scope clearly distinguish the nature of advanced practice for ANP beyond generalist nursing practice (e.g. advanced and more in-depth education and critical thinking)?
- Are there regulations and policies in place or being discussed to support these advanced roles and functions as described in the scope of practice?

(Adapted from Schober and Affara [55])

In providing a model for developing scope, standards, policies, and procedures (SSPP) Jhpiego [34] provides guiding commentary on developing a scope of practice:

> Scopes of practice form the foundation of a health professional's designated work... [and] are vital because they inform which standards and competencies are identified, communicate role expectations, inform curriculum content and practice standards, assist with making skill-mix decisions, and assist with introducing more coherence in the process of health workforce planning (p.1).

In the SSPP model, scope, standards, policies, and procedures are linked with one being the foundation for another. Professional standards develop from the defined scope of practice of a profession. The scope of practice distinguishes the professional's range of activities – roles, functions, responsibilities, accountability, authority, and decision-making capacity. This model proposes that following a situational and task analysis categories of personnel with their scopes are defined, and competencies and standards are established and then operationalized. This model provides a broad country based proposal with an aim to promote coherence and relevance to inform delivery of healthcare services. Refer to Chap. 6, Professional Regulation, for further discussion and a figure depicting the SSPP model as it relates to development of professional regulations (see Figure 6.1).

When considering models and strategies defining scope of practice for the APN, difficulty arises when there is resistance to move beyond a generalist nurse definition to develop standards that emphasize the knowledge, competencies, level of clinical judgment and decision making that APNs bring to their practice setting. In settings with highly specialized APN roles, a specific scope may be developed that builds on and is consistent with a more generic APN scope of practice. In countries or regions where there is no legal or published scope of practice for ANP, practice guidelines are based on the best fit for the circumstances dictated by the country's particular situation in respect to healthcare services. This approach suggests a broad and flexible method of defining a professional scope of practice. Controversial issues that may arise in developing the APN scope of practice are discussed in Sects. 3.4.1, 3.4.2, and 3.4.3.

3.4 Controversial Issues

Survey findings [18, 50, 52] and descriptions of country profiles of ANP development (see Chap. 2) demonstrate diversity in description and function of APNs. Topics such as prescriptive authority, establishing an initial diagnosis by an APN, the granting of hospital privileges to allow the APN to admit to hospitals, and authority to refer to other services and/or healthcare professionals raises areas of disagreement depending on the setting or country where the debate takes place. Prescriptive authority, making the initial clinical diagnosis, and obtaining hospital privileges for the APN are discussed next. Points to consider when exploring inclusion of these options in the APN scope of practice are suggested.

3.4.1 Prescriptive Authority

When discussing ANP, debate focuses on changes in the boundaries of nursing practice and the impact of this change on other healthcare professions. One concern is that expanded nursing practice will impinge on the professional role of physicians [3]. Prescriptive authority for nurses, nurse prescribing, or medicine management is one issue that fuels animated debate. Literature suggests that physicians are critical of nurse prescribing, asserting that nurses simply do not have the knowledge to prescribe medicines correctly [10, 37, 38]. Even though the center of attention is on the appropriateness of nurse prescribing, investigation of the realities of nursing practice reveals that at times nurses are already safely prescribing but outside a legal framework and without appropriate education supportive of current practice. Furthermore, prescriptive authority would seem to be a prerequisite for some APN roles, such as a nurse practitioner practicing in primary care, to reach its full potential. When aligned with the concept of ANP, prescribing can be defined "as the steps of information gathering, clinical decision making, communication, and evaluation which results in the initiation, continuation or cessation of a medicine" (Cashin et al. [14], p.8)

Even though nurse prescribing is a contentious issue, there is an identified increase in the numbers of countries where nurse are legally permitted to prescribe medicines [4, 37, 38]. Ball [4] noted this growth by referring to examples of six countries with nurse prescribing that are mentioned in the 2000 ICN monograph on nurse prescribing [9]. The noted number increased to 10 in 2004 [10] and then 16 in 2009 [4] indicating a growing trend in relation to prescriptive authority within nursing practice.

Nurse prescribing is often associated with APN roles; however, levels of prescriptive authority vary from country to country and can be affiliated with general nursing practice, not necessarily with ANP. There is little consistency reported across countries as to what capacity nurses have in prescribing [4, 10, 37, 38]. Therefore, a key question that arises is not "Can nurses prescribe?" but "To what extent is nurse prescribing established?" (Ball [4], p. 67).

As ANP evolves internationally it is possible there will be an increasing link of prescriptive authority to APN roles as demonstrated in a 2014 requirement in New Zealand where prior to 1 July 2014 it had been possible to register as a either a prescribing or nonprescribing nurse practitioner (NP). Since 1 July 2014, the nurse practitioner scope of practice stipulates that the group of NPs unauthorized to prescribe "must not prescribe as an authorized prescriber (nurse practitioner)." Prescribing pathways in New Zealand facilitate the transition from nonprescribing NP status to achieving prescribing authority with the choice of one of two pathways:

- Qualifications that include a pharmacology course and a prescribing practicum requiring 100 h of supervised prescribing practice and competence assessment by a medical mentor or nurse practitioner
- or
- Nurse practitioners without the appropriate qualification must complete a Nursing Council approved pharmacology paper and a prescribing practicum that includes 100 h of supervised prescribing practice and a competence assessment by a medical practitioner and a nurse practitioner or supply a portfolio that demonstrates the equivalent knowledge and skills plus complete a panel review.

(Nursing Council of New Zealand [48])

Changes to the Medicines Amendment ACT 2013 named nurse practitioners and optometrists as authorized prescribers. This change enables NPs to prescribe all medicines appropriate to their scope of practice, rather than limiting them to a specific list of medicines. This change recognized the safe and appropriate prescribing practice of nurse practitioners over the previous 9 years and is expected to:

- Improve patient access to timely care
- Make best use of the skills of the nurse practitioner workforce
- Reduce patient cost

(New Zealand Ministry of Health 2016).

In looking at seven country and regional examples that have realized nurse prescribing (Australia, Canada, Ireland, New Zealand, Sweden, the UK, the USA), Kroezen et al. [37] noted that prescribing at some level has been in place in the USA since the 1960s, whereas it is a relatively new phenomenon in most other countries. Community nurses in the UK started prescribing in 1998, subsequently two other models of prescribing were introduced followed in 2002 by "independent prescribing" then "supplementary prescribing" in 2003. Prescriptive authority for nurses in Canada, New Zealand, and the USA followed the development of the APN role. Nurse prescribing in Sweden was initiated independent of an ANP presence. All Western-European and Anglo-Saxon countries that have initiated nurse prescribing have placed legal restrictions on which categories of nurses can prescribe and under what conditions they are allowed to prescribe. Regulation occurs at a national, state, or regional level depending on the country. In addition to defined formularies for medicines, protocols are used to restrict independent nurse prescribing.

Four models of nurse prescribing have been proposed in ICN monographs [4, 10]: independent authority, dependent/collaborative authority, group protocol/patient care directives, and time and dose prescribing or patient specific protocols (Refer to Fig. 3.3). Kroezen et al. [37] in an analysis of the literature from Western and Anglo-Saxon countries identified three models (independent prescribing, supplementary/collaborative prescribing, patient group directives) similar to the ICN models. However, these researchers took note of the ICN models for nurse prescribing but did not consider "time and dose prescribing" as a form of nurse prescribing as nurses are only allowed to alter particular medications usually prescribed by a physician.

The manner in which nurse prescribing has evolved is shaped by the motivation to identify this as a nursing component in the context of the country. Without a clear necessity and supportive infrastructure, promotion of nurse prescribing may fail to succeed. Conversely a shortage of physicians, an emergent healthcare crises, or difficulty delivering healthcare services can be the stimulus needed regardless of a supportive infrastructure, education, or legislation [4]. Key elements identified as significant in progressing to the promotion of nurse prescribing include:

- A clear need
- Legislation/regulation to support practice
- Ability of nursing to participate in and influence the policy process regulating prescribing
- Evidence of cost effectiveness

(Adapted from Ball [4], pp.71–72)

In addition, based on a review of country cases, Ball [4] suggests that the following factors influence the extent to which nurse prescribing is implemented:

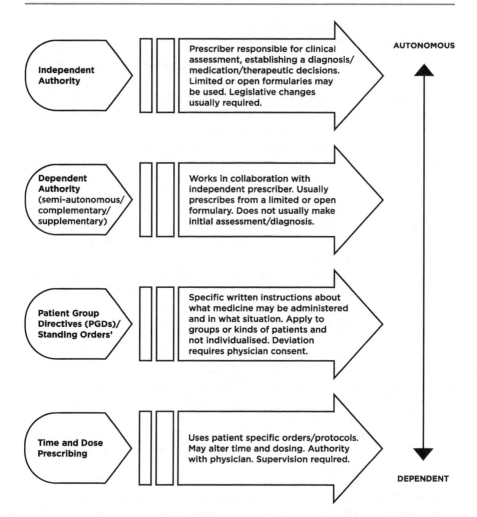

Fig. 3.3   Models of nurse prescribing (Ball [4], Kroezen et al. [37], Schober and Affara [55])

- The time to develop regulation/education to prepare nurses qualified to prescribe especially if prescribing is restricted to master's prepared nurses
- Resource issues such that the public does not incur increase costs for prescriptions written by nurses
- State/regional variation especially in situations where prescriptive authority is dependent on medical approval
- National political will in the face of opposition from other professions
- Limited or restrictive formularies
- Lack of research to evaluate prescriptive practices by nurses (Ball [4], pp 69–70)

The exact nature of nurse prescribing internationally varies significantly from circumstances where nurses prescribe independently to situations where prescriptive authority is restricted under close supervision of a physician. Most often the jurisdiction for prescribing is based on the authority of the medical profession to influence mechanisms in select countries that have led to nurse prescribing. Even though an increase in nurse prescribing has been noted, especially in association with ANP, further research is needed to substantiate this presence and resultant outcomes.

3.4.2 The Diagnosis Debate

Making an initial diagnostic decision can be viewed as informed and educated decision-making by a healthcare professional with and on behalf of a patient or family [55]. In some settings, the APN scope of practice can be excessively restricted when the ability to make a diagnosis is relegated only to medicine, especially in primary care settings. For APNs, in roles where they are making an initial diagnosis for illness accompanied by a therapeutic management plan, the scope of practice is likely to overlap with decision-making traditionally associated with medicine versus a nursing diagnosis that is considered as a plan that follows and is somewhat separate from the initial diagnosis. Conversation related to initial diagnoses by an APN brings up the following themes for discussion:

- Identification of diagnostic capability within ANP scope of practice
- Definition of the circumstances or setting where an APN can make an initial or differential diagnosis
- Examination of the authority needed for an APN to make a diagnosis as well as ordering and interpreting diagnostic testing

Investigation of the topic of diagnosis as it relates to APN practice warrants a review of practice acts of other healthcare professionals within a setting or country. Some practice acts relegate making an initial diagnosis along with examining a patient only to physicians. In the USA as the nurse practitioner (NP) role in primary care evolved and adopted a medical model for diagnosing, a perspective transpired that NPs were "stepping over the invisible medical boundary" away from a nursing model into a sphere claimed by physicians (Cockerham and Keeling [16], p. 17). Over time with increased education, legislation, and an increasing NP presence this attitude has become less prevalent. Just as the subject of prescriptive authority stimulates heated discussions, dialogue on a scope of practice for APN that includes an APN making an initial diagnosis requires deliberation based on country context. It is the view of the author that using a common diagnostic language and approach is one way to attain consistency of care in provision of healthcare services.

3.4.3 Hospital Privileges

The authority to admit to and discharge from a healthcare facility has traditionally been associated with physicians in many parts of the world. There is an increasing recognition that these policies have the potential to compromise efficient and effective healthcare delivery. The term hospital privileges originated from the process of awarding a status to physicians who had successfully completed a hospital's screening process. According to hospital policy, healthcare professionals with approved privileges have full access to records of patients they admit, decision-making authority over management within the institution as well as readiness for discharge [12].

Obtaining hospital privileges allows APNs to provide specific care or treatment in a particular institutional setting. Privileges are usually granted based on license, education, training, experience, competence, health status, and judgment. The American Nurses Association developed a multifaceted strategy to address barriers in the USA and ensure that APNs can obtain appropriate clinical privileges [60]. The possibility to be credentialed as full members of a hospital medical staff, with admitting, discharge, and appropriate clinical privileges is viewed as essential to practice for many APNs [6]. Even though the urgency of this issue is not high on the international healthcare agenda, the vibrant nature of healthcare reform could encourage healthcare planners to see this choice as advantageous for APNs and the populations they care for.

3.5   Competencies and Advanced Practice

Regardless of role preparation, identifying competencies is one method for assessing accountability [26]. This section introduces the idea of competencies and their link to scope of practice for the APN. Chapter 4, Education, provides a further discussion of core competencies, competency statements, and identification of competencies that provide a foundation for ANP education.

Competence can be viewed as an appraisal of performance, a point of reference, an element of professional practice, or a defined stage of professional achievement:

> A level of performance demonstrating the effective application of knowledge, skill and judgment (Styles and Affara [59], p. 44)

Developing standards and competency guidelines has long been a key element of the work of the International Council of Nurses in an effort to clarify nursing's role and scope of practice in relation to healthcare [26]. In 2003, a framework was developed to establish the competencies of the generalist nurse along with an implementation model suggesting steps to link competencies to country context [29, 30], The concepts that make up the ICN framework for the generalist nurse also form the basis for the ICN APN framework [32]. The connection between the generalist nurse and the APN is the common core that links these two disciplines.

The degree of critical thinking, skills, knowledge, and accountability increases between the education of the generalist nurse and the APN. Even though the range and depth of practice is gained "through additional education and experience in clinical practice; the core does not change and it remains the context of nursing" (ICN [32], p. 9). The original ICN framework for the generalist nurse was revised and updated in 2008 [31] and a schematic image is included in the APN document [32].

Even though competencies are widely used in describing APN roles, the practice of determining and assigning suitable role competencies is contentious. Literature suggests that the universal acceptance of this guiding principle is not substantiated by reliable evidence and is problematic in differentiating dissimilar levels of competence [24, 61]. Despite discrepancies and controversies in their usefulness, the application of this concept occupies the attention of regulatory authorities as a way to demonstrate the safety of APNs. Lacking a better alternative, the identification of competencies will likely continue to be used to measure and standardize ANP.

Advanced skills are one component of APN competencies. Section 3.5.1 differentiates between advanced tasks or skills and advanced critical thinking.

3.5.1 Advanced Tasks Versus Advanced Critical Thinking

The ability to develop a perspective of advanced roles beyond simply performing advanced tasks is a critical component of ANP and promotes APN roles that are nursing-centered as well as advanced in practice. It is the depth of decision-making and critical thinking associated with clinical reasoning that distinguishes the APN from the generalist nurse and the RN specialist. Advanced tasks are components of the scope of practice but are not the essence of ANP. Fundamentals of ANP originate from a "philosophy of autonomous nursing practice and accountability for that practice" (Bowling and Stilwell [5], p. 21). Carryer [13] stressed that a professional viewpoint guides the principles and nature of practice for ANP, not defined tasks. New and advanced tasks are valid components of ANP when they offer ease, comprehensiveness, and continuity in provision of healthcare services.

3.5.2 Task Reallocation and Task Shifting

The World Health Organization (WHO) in response to critical shortages of healthcare professionals considered "task shifting" as an intervention that showed potential for strengthening delivery of healthcare services by rearranging the skill mix within a country's healthcare system [62, 64]. Task shifting refers to:

- Shifting tasks from one category of healthcare worker to another
- Shifting tasks to a new category of healthcare worker developed to meet specific healthcare goals

Concepts of "skill mix" or "skills substitution" [11, 57] have also been suggested to meet the workforce challenges for healthcare delivery suggesting models similar to the proposed WHO intervention. Since the time of the WHO publications [62, 64], even though the process seems logical, the terminology "task shifting" has been challenged as hierarchical based on physician-centered care that is seen to have decreasing contemporary relevance. This premise was commented on at the XIX International AIDS Conference in Washington D.C. and it was suggested that needs based task-sharing or team based care would be better designed to enable diverse health professionals to achieve their full potential [49]. Although the reallocating of tasks and service delivery is not specific to ANP, the concept is frequently discussed and impacts how service delivery by nurses is viewed in relation to other healthcare workers.

The literature on task shifting in Sub-Saharan Africa demonstrates comparable outcomes for physician or nurse led care [35]. Many African countries are increasingly taking on approaches of "task-shifting" or the delegating of tasks upwards or downwards through the perceived hierarchies of the healthcare professions in order to address health workforce shortages [63]. However, debate on task shifting and medical substitution in Africa appears to be developing quite independently from discussion on advanced nursing practice despite the potential overlap between the two ideas [20, 21, 56]. A survey of nursing and midwifery regulatory reform in east, central, and southern Africa concluded that there is a lack of alignment between the regulatory environment and the expanding role of nurses [42]. East et al. [21] propose that the potential contribution of APNs to Kenyan healthcare goes beyond policies of task- shifting where nurses substitute for physicians. Increased recognition and support for practice development and leadership functions of APNs while strengthening their expertise in clinical practice is suggested.

A study conducted in the Netherlands [36] commissioned by the Dutch Ministry of Health investigated task reallocation for nurse specialists (NS) and physician assistants (PA). Study findings indicated variations in how reallocation took place from medicine to the NS or PA and revealed financial and/or structural restrictions as to how task reallocation occurred. Despite obstacles and restrictions to practice, these two categories of healthcare professionals commenced to effectively perform medical tasks in the interest of quality and integrated care. Tasks were seen as substitutes or supplementary to the physician and transferred to the NS or PA to allow the physician to concentrate on more complex healthcare issues.

The author offers the topic of task reallocation or task shifting for debate and discussion as professionals, healthcare planners, and policymakers address the comprehensive nature of the world's healthcare needs. The reality of this view of healthcare delivery and a view of task shifting as it is linked to ANP remains unclear and likely to be country specific depending on critical healthcare needs. Focusing excessively on only task based duties for the APN could be seen as restrictive to the full potential of the capacity of this nursing role. The inclusion of ANP competencies that are viewed as only tasks needs to be addressed clearly and directly in a well developed scope of practice. A *Joint Health Professions Statement* by WHO [65] on task shifting emphasized the need for adequate planning and monitoring to avoid a fragmented and disjointed approach that fails to meet the identified aims of task shifting, task reallocation, and skill mix.

Conclusion

This chapter explores the diverse nature of advanced nursing practice. When considering the introduction and development of advanced nursing, no single approach or definition includes all aspects of these varied roles, especially in the beginning stages. Essential characteristics and basic assumptions of advanced practice nursing are highlighted. Country and regional illustrations described in Chap. 2 demonstrate that changes supportive of ANP take place over years and decades of decision-making under diverse and complex circumstances. This chapter takes note of these country profiles and builds on that knowledge emphasizing that inclusion of new nursing roles such as APNs must be tailored to country needs, healthcare context, and resource capabilities.

References

1. American Association of Nurse Practitioners (AANP) (2015a) Use of terms such as mid-level provider and physician extender, Position Statements and Papers, Retrieved on 7 Mar 2016 from https://www.aanp.org/publications/position-statements-papers
2. American Association of Nurse Practitioners (AANP) (2015b) Scope of practice for nurse practitioners, Position Statements and Papers, Retrieved on 7 Mar 2016 from https://www.aanp.org/publications/position-statements-papers
3. Baird A (2001) Diagnosis and prescribing: the impact of nurse prescribing on professional roles. Primary Health Care 11:24–26
4. Ball J (2009) Implementing nurse prescribing: an update review current practice internationally. Monograph 25. International Council of Nurses, Geneva
5. Bowling A, Stilwell B (eds) (1988) The nurse in family practice: practice nurses and nurse practitioners in primary health care. Scutari Press, London
6. Brassard A, Smolenski M (2011) Removing barriers to advanced practice nurse care: hospital privileges. Insight on the issues, Issues 55, September. American Association of Retired Persons Public Policy Institute, Washington, DC
7. Brown SJ (1998) A framework for advanced practice nursing. J Prof Nurs 14(3):157–164
8. Bryant-Lukosius D, DiCenso A (2004) A framework for the introduction and evaluation of advanced practice nursing roles. J Adv Nurs 48(5):530–540
9. Buchan J, Calman L (2000) Implementing nurse prescribing: an update review current practice internationally. International Council of Nurses, Geneva
10. Buchan J, Calman L (2004) Implementing nurse prescribing: an update review current practice internationally. Monograph 16. International Council of Nurses, Geneva
11. Buchan J, Dal Poz MR (2002) Skill mix in the health care workforce: reviewing the evidence. Bull World Health Organization 80(7):575–80. Access: https://www.who.int/hrh/documents/skill_mix.pdf
12. Buppert C (2015) Nurse practitioner's business practice and legal guide, 5th edn. Jones & Bartlett Learning, Burlington
13. Carryer J (2002) Nurse practitioners: an evolutionary role. Kai Taiki Nursing New Zealand 8(10):23

14. Cashin A, Buckley T, Donoghue J, Heartfield M, Bryce J, Cox, Gosby H, Kelly J, Dunn S (2015) Development of the nurse practitioner standards for practice. Policy Polit Nurs Pract 0(0):1–11. doi:10.1177/152715584233
15. Clark J, Lang N (1992) Nursing's next advance: an internal classification for nursing practice. Int Nurs Rev 39(4):109–111, p128
16. Cockerham AZ, Keeling AW (2014) A brief history of advanced practice nursing in the United States. In: Hamric AB, Hanson CM, Tracy MF, O'Grady ET (eds) Advanced practice nursing: an integrative approach, 5th edn. Elsevier Saunders, St. Louis, pp 1–26
17. Coleman S, Fox J (2003) Clinical practice benchmarking and advanced practice. In: McGee P, Castledine G (eds) Advanced nursing practice, 2nd edn. Blackwell Publishing, Oxford, pp 47–58
18. Delemaire M, LaFortune G (2010) Nurses in advanced roles: a description and evaluation of experiences in 12 developed countries. OECD Health Working Papers, No. 54, OECD Publishing. doi:10.1787/5kmbrcfms5g7-en
19. DiCenso A, Bryant-Lukosius D, Bourgeault I, Martin-Misener R, Donald F, Abelson J, Kaasalainen S, Kilpatrick K, Kioke S, Carter N, Harbman P (2010) Clinical nurse specialists and nurse practitioners in Canada: a decision support synthesis. Canadian Health Services Research Foundation, Ottawa
20. Donald F, Bryant-Lukosius D, Martin-Misener R, Kaasalainen S, Kilpatrick K, Carter N, Harbman P, Bourgeault I, DiCenso A (2010) Clinical nurse specialists and nurse practitioners: title confusion and lack of role clarity. Can J Nurs Leadersh Nurs Leadersh 23(Special Issue):189–210
21. Duffield C, Gardner G, Chang A, Catling-Paull C (2009) Advanced nursing practice: a global perspective. Collegian 16(2):55–62
22. East LA, Arudo J, Loefler M, Evans CM (2014) Exploring the potential for advanced nursing practice role development in Kenya: a qualitative study. BMC Nurs 13:33
23. Gardner G, Carryer J, Dunn S, Gardner A (2004) Nurse practitioner Standards Project: Report to Australian Nursing and Midwifery Council. Australian Nursing and Midwifery Council
24. Gardner G, Chang A, Duffield C (2007) Making nursing work: Breaking through the role confusion of advanced practice nursing. J Adv Nurs 57:382–391. doi:10.1111/j.1365-2648.2007.04114x
25. Girot E (2000) Assessment of graduates and diplomats in practice in the UK – are we measuring the same level of competence? J Clin Nurs 9:330–337
26. Gordon SE (1989) Accountability in nursing: a many-faceted concept. In: Leddy S, Pepper JM (eds) Conceptual bases of professional nursing, 2nd edn. Lippincott, Philadelphia
27. Hamric AB (1996) A definition of advanced practice nursing. In: Hamric AB, Spross JA, Hanson CA (eds) Advanced nursing practice: an integrative approach. WB Saunders, Philadelphia, pp 25–41
28. Hancock C (2004) Unity with diversity: ICN's framework of competencies. Guest Editorial. J Adv Nurs 47(2):119
29. Hanson CM (2014) Understanding regulatory, legal and credentialing requirements. In: Hamric AB, Hanson CM, Tracy MF, O'Grady ET (eds) Advanced practice nursing: an integrative approach. Elsevier Saunders, St. Louis, pp 557–578
30. International Council of Nursing (ICN) (2002) Definition and characteristics of the role. Retrieved 9 Mar 2016 from http://www.icn-apnetwork.org
31. International Council of Nursing (ICN) (2003) Framework of competencies for the generalist nurse. ICN, Geneva
32. International Council of Nursing (ICN) (2003) An implementation model for the ICN framework of competencies for the generalist nurse. ICN, Geneva
33. International Council of Nurses (ICN) (2008) Nursing care continuum – framework and competencies, ICN regulation series. International Council of Nurses, Geneva
34. International Council of Nurses (ICN) (2008) The scope of practice, standards and competencies of the advanced practice nurse, ICN regulation series. International Council of Nurses, Geneva

35. International Council of Nurses (ICN) (2009) Framework of competencies for the nurse specialist, ICN regulation series. International Council of Nurses, Geneva
36. Jhpiego (2016) Scope, standards, policies and procedures model. Retrieved on 8 Mar 2016 from https://reprolineplus.org/system/files/resources/03_SSPP%20Model_tc.pdf
37. Holzemer B (2008) Building a qualified global workforce. Int Nurs Rev 55(3):241–242
38. Kouwen AJ, van den Brink GTWJ (2014) Task reallocation and cost prices: Research of obstacles concerning substitution. Report from Radboud University Medical Center to the Dutch Ministry of Health, Welfare and Sport
39. Kroezen M, van Dijk L, Groenewegen PP, Francke AL (2011) Nurse prescribing of medicines in Western European and Anglo-Saxon countries: a systematic review of the literature. BMC Health Serv Res 11:127, http://www.biomedcentral/1472-6963/11/127
40. Latter S, Courtenay M (2004) Effectiveness of nurse prescribing: a review of the literature. J Clin Nurs 13:26–32. doi:10.1046/j.1365-2702.2003.00839.x
41. Jones ML (2005) Role development and effective practice in specialist and advanced practice roles in acute hospital settings: systematic review and meta-synthesis. J Adv Nurs 49(2):191–2009
42. Lewandowski W, Adamic K (2009) Substantive areas of clinical nurse specialist practice. A comprehensive review of the literature. Clin Nurs Spec J Adv Nurs Pract 23:73–92. doi:10.1097/NUR.0b013e31819971d0
43. Mantzoukas S, Watkinson S (2007) Review of advanced nursing practice: the international literature and developing the generic features. J Clin Nurs 16:28–37
44. McCarthy C, Voss J, Salmon M, Gross J, Kelley M, Riley P (2013) Nursing and midwifery regulatory reform in east, central and southern Africa: a survey of key stakeholders. Human Res Health 11(29) doi:10.1186/1478-4491-11-29
45. McGee P (2009) The conceptualisation of advanced practice. In: McGee P (ed) Advanced practice in nursing and the allied health professions, 3rd edn. Wiley-Blackwell, The Atrium, Southern Gate, Chichester, pp 43–56
46. National Association of Clinical Nurse Specialists (NACNS) (2016) Statement on APRN consensus model implementation. NACNS, Washington, DC, Accessed 26 April 2016 from http://www.nacns.org/docs/NACNSConsensusModel.pdf
47. Nursing Council of New Zealand (NCNZ) (2014) Nurse practitioner scope *of* practice: Guidelines for applicants. Accessed 7 Mar 2016 from http://www.nursingcouncil.org.nz/Nurses/Scopes-of-practice/Nurse-practitioner
48. New Zealand Ministry of Health (2014) 1 July 2014 changes to prescribing, Accessed 7 Mar 2016 from http://www.health.govt.nz/our-work/regulation-health-and-disability-system/1-july-2014-changes-prescribing
49. Olson D (2012) Task sharing, not task shifting: team approach is best for HIV Care. Access from http://www.capacityplus.org/task-sharing-not-task-shifting
50. Pulcini J, Jelic M, Gul R, Loke AY (2010) An international survey on advanced practice nursing education, practice and regulation. J Nurs Scholarsh 42(1):31–39
51. Roberts-Davis M, Read S (2001) Clinical role clarification: using the Delphi method to establish similarities and differences between nurse practitioners and clinical nurse specialists. J Clin Nurs 10(1):33–43
52. Sastre-Fullana P, De Pedro-Gomez JE, Bennasar-Veny M, Serrano-Gallardo P, Morales-Ascencio JM (2014) Competency frameworks for advanced practice nursing: a literature review. Int Nurs Rev 61(4):534–542
53. Schober M (2004) Advanced practice nursing: perspectives and challenges. Nursing Excellence in Transactions (NET), 8th Issue. Queen Elizabeth Hospital, Central Nursing Division, Hong Kong
54. Schober M (2013) Factors Influencing the Development of Advanced Practice Nursing in Singapore. Doctoral thesis, Sheffield Hallam University, Sheffield Hallam University archives. Accessed 5 Mar 2016 from http://shura.shu.ac.uk/7799/
55. Schober M, Affara F (2006) Advanced nursing practice. Blackwell Publishing, Oxford

56. Shumbusho F, van Griensven J, Lowrance D, Turate I, Weaver M, Price J, Binagwaho A (2009) Task shifting for scale-up of HIV care: evaluation of nurse-centered antiretroviral treatment at rural health centers in Rwanda. PLoS Med 6(10), e1000163. doi:10.1371/journal. pmed.1000163
57. Sibbald B, Chen J, McBride A (2004) Changing the skill-mix of the healthcare Workforce. J Health Serv Res Policy 9(Suppl 1):28–38
58. Spross JA (2014) Conceptualizations of advanced practice nursing. In: Hamric AB, Hanson CM, Tracy MF, O'Grady ET (eds) Advanced practice nursing: an integrative approach. Elsevier, St. Louis, pp 27–66
59. Styles MM, Affara FA (1997) ICN on regulation: towards 21st century models. ICN, Geneva
60. Summers L (2016) Clinical privileges: Opening the doors for APRNs. The American Nurse. American Nurses Association, Silver Spring, Maryland
61. Watson R, Stimpson A, Topping A, Porock D (2002) Clinical competence assessment in nursing: a systematic review of the literature. J Adv Nurs 39(5):421–431
62. World Health Organization (WHO) (2006) Working together for health: the World Health Report 2006. WHO, Geneva. Accessible from http://www.who.int/whr/2006.whr06_en.pdf
63. World Health Organization (WHO) (2007) Task shifting to tackle health worker shortages. Accessible from http://www.who.int/healthsystems/task_shifting_booklet.pdf
64. World Health Organization (WHO) (2008) Task shifting: rational distribution of tasks among health workforce teams: global recommendations and guidelines. WHO, Geneva
65. World Health Professions Alliance (2008) Joint health professions statement on task shifting. Accessible from http://www.whpa.org/statement_12_principles.pdf

Education

4

Abstract

The credibility of Advanced Nursing Practice is based on the educational preparation that the advanced practice nurse receives. Defining educational preparation at an advanced level provides a basis to differentiate advanced practice from that of the generalist and specialist nurse while also building on basic nursing education. This chapter describes and discusses core issues to consider when developing or refining a program. Topics include program planning, curriculum design, teaching methods, criteria for student selection, and qualifying requirements for faculty/staff/student preceptors. Emphasis is placed on reaching a decision on the role and function expected of the APN in the healthcare workforce linking expected role competencies to the planning of an educational course or program. It is not within the scope of this chapter to provide in-depth coverage of all aspects for ANP education but to discuss the essential principles to consider.

Keywords

Program planning • Curriculum design • Student criteria • Teaching methods • Qualified educators • Preceptors

The credibility of Advanced Nursing Practice is based on the educational preparation that the advanced practice nurse receives. Defining educational preparation at an advanced level provides a basis to differentiate advanced practice from that of the generalist and specialist nurse while also building on basic nursing education. This chapter describes and discusses core issues to consider when developing or refining a program. Topics include program planning, curriculum design, teaching methods, criteria for student selection, and qualifying requirements for faculty/staff/student preceptors. Emphasis is placed on reaching a decision on the role and function expected of the APN in the healthcare workforce linking expected role competencies to the planning of an educational course or program. It is not within the scope of this chapter to provide in-depth coverage of all aspects for ANP education but to discuss the essential principles to consider.

© Springer International Publishing Switzerland 2016

M. Schober, *Introduction to Advanced Nursing Practice*,

DOI 10.1007/978-3-319-32204-9_4

4.1   Characteristics of Advanced Nursing Practice Education

Education beyond the preparation of the generalist nurse is critical in providing a
sound basis for preparation of a nurse for the APN role. Pulcini et al. [24] in conducting an international survey found that education varies widely from short certificate or diploma courses to graduate degrees. However, the survey demonstrated
that Increasingly ANP education is occurring at a master's level. ICN [14] suggests
standards to consider when developing educational programs for ANP and recommended master's education as entry level into practice. The ICN guidelines include
the following:

- Programs prepare the student, a registered/licensed nurse, for practice beyond that of
  a generalist nurse by including opportunities to access knowledge and skills as well
  as demonstrate its integration in clinical practice as a safe, competent and autonomous practitioner
- Programs prepare the authorized nurse to practice within the nation's healthcare
  system to the full extent of the role as set out in the scope of practice
- Programs are staffed by nursing faculty who are qualified and prepared at or beyond
  the level of the student undertaking the program of study
- Programs are accredited/approved by the authorized national or international credentialing body
- Programs facilitate lifelong learning and maintenance of competencies
- Programs provide students access to a sufficient range of clinical experience to apply
  and consolidate, under supervision, [information learned in] the theoretical course
  content

                                                                            (ICN [14], p. 21)

   Issues impacting ANP education are multifactoral. Educators and program
planners undertake matters from designing a curriculum to envisioning resources
needed for long-term sustainability. Challenges include seeking financial resources,
recruiting qualified educators, selecting appropriate clinical sites, identifying men-
tors/role models, and planning a suitably balanced program linked to identified
competencies for APN practice. National nursing associations, regulatory authorities, governmental agencies, and academic institutions will likely have a say in the
establishment of the standards for ANP education that in turn contribute to legiti-
matizing the APN roles.

4.1.1   Identifying Competencies: A Guide for Education
            Development

Identified APN competencies focuses on the outcome of a learning experience and
refers to the performance of the practitioner [26]. Competencies refer to the ability
of an APN to do something to a defined standard with core competencies expected
of all students upon completion of an educational program for entry into practice.
Chapter 3 introduces the topic of competence as it relates to APN practice. This section focuses on the topic of competencies and its relevance to ANP education.

Hamric [12] suggests that direct clinical care is the central competency for ANP that informs all others. Six additional competencies are mentioned that are viewed to further define ANP "regardless of role function or setting" and are as follows:

- Guidance and coaching
- Consultation
- Evidence-based practice
- Leadership
- Collaboration
- Ethical decision-making

(Hamric [12], p. 76)

Each of the competencies is defined in relation to the context where the APN expects to practice. Students do not graduate fully prepared in all competencies but will strive to develop an interaction of competencies over time. It is not the intent of the author to elaborate on extensive details of each competency but to depict the complexity of how competencies are identified for ANP. Achieving the expected competencies is acquired through supervised and mentored/precepted experiences emphasizing the development of analytical skills. These skills are the basis for evaluating and providing evidenced-based patient-centered healthcare services that include advanced knowledge of healthcare delivery.

4.2   Variations in Educational Philosophy and Approach

Setting master's level education as a goal for ANP preparation is an international trend [14, 24] aligned also with a bachelor's degree required by many countries as entry level into the nursing profession. In initial stages of planning and development, graduate education may be a goal to strive for in refining an educationalist approach for ANP. Scarce financial and human resources, limited opportunities for advanced nursing education, shortage of qualified nursing educators, and lack of recognition of nursing as a profession detract from the likelihood of reaching this criterion immediately. When no APNs or APN models exist in the country, human resources may include expert nurses with extensive experience along with medical consultants and other healthcare professionals able to lend their expertise (e.g., pharmacy). Coordination of diverse expert resources can guide the educationalist foundation until a presence of APNs and qualified nursing educators is established. Competing priorities on a country's healthcare or workforce agenda may dictate a need to set graduate level ANP education as a standard to attain as plans evolve and education strategies progress.

In describing nurse practitioner development in the United States [28] noted that over time education evolved from a postregistered nurse certificate to master's degree level. Medical schools, hospitals, and schools of nursing commonly offered continued education options initially. Educational progress evolved in response to healthcare needs and educational developments. Curricula has become more refined and standardized as to content and clinical requirements [3]. Based on recommendations from professional associations, entry level education for ANP has, for the most part, progressed to Doctor of Nursing Practice (DNP) [2] in the country.

In Botswana in 1981, the Institute of Health Sciences (IHS) established a Family Nurse Practitioner diploma program that focused on primary healthcare [27]. Originally designed as 1 year of study the program progressed to 18 months and in 2007/2008 established a four-semester format. In addition, the University of Botswana offers a master's of nursing degree that includes an advanced practice clinical choice. It is hoped that the two programs will develop greater "program articulation" to allow students or graduates from the IHS program to enter the master's program at the University of Botswana [23]. Similarly, in an effort to meet country healthcare needs and with support of the World Health Organization, a 1-year Advanced Diploma of Nursing was established in 1992 in Samoa for post-basic training to enhance clinical assessment and decision-making skills of experienced nurses as community-based nurse practitioners [31].

In contrast to an evolving approach to ANP education over time, New Zealand's framework [21] for nurse practitioner endorsement established a requirement of a clinically focused master's education, or its equivalent, for entry level to practice at the start of the initiative. Updated requirements [22] continue to require an NCNZ approved clinical master's degree program that includes demonstration of advanced practice competencies. Likewise, APN education at the National University of Singapore was launched from the start as a Master of Science in Nursing (MScN) degree in 2003. Prior to this time, the only option for a graduate degree or ANP preparation was to complete a study out of the country. The MScN education program for APNs has been successful in attracting students from Singapore and with its success has expanded specialty options [25].

Canada presents a situation of dual roles using advanced nursing practice as the umbrella term (clinical nurse specialist [CNS] & nurse practitioner [NP]). As a result, the country has a history of dual levels of education. The hospital-based CNSs have been educated mainly at the graduate level since the 1980s. Education for NPs, who practice mainly in primary health care settings, has been uneven ranging from a postbaccalaureate diploma in some jurisdictions to a master's degree in others [16]. Arguments supporting a graduate level degree for all NPs in Canada have been proposed; however, access to this level of education in rural and remote areas of the country is a continuing concern [18].

Illustrations of variance in country philosophy and approach to ANP education highlight the influence of regional and country contexts. In developing an educationalist program, it is important to start with a curriculum- or competency-based framework relevant to the expected function of the APN. The following section discusses planning a curriculum and creating a curriculum design.

4.3   Curriculum Development

When planning curricula for ANP defining basic elements of the projected content and level of education is key. The current status of education for the generalist nurse in the country should be taken into account. Since ANP education builds on the foundation of education in place for the generalist nurse, program planners need to consider what knowledge and skills the student will need to acquire to transit to an advanced level of practice including in an area of specialized practice. Content based on and linked to the definition defined scope of practice and identified competencies for the expected APN roles form the basis for understandable and sustainable curriculum goals. Nurse educators designing curricula should have the qualifications, expertise, and have an understanding of the APN scope of practice to take on program development and curriculum design in order to establish relevant requirements for ANP education.

4.3.1   Curriculum Framework

Utilizing a curriculum framework as a guide is helpful in identifying key components to consider in curriculum planning. A suggested framework based on three conceptual cornerstones – curriculum goals, healthcare needs, and health policy – is represented in Fig. 4.1 [10]. The flow of the framework promotes a continuous interface between the three cornerstones allowing for adjustments and adaptation to the country setting and respective healthcare environments. It should be noted that describing role definition, scope of practice, and APN competencies are the foundation for identifying curriculum goals. (See Chap. 3 for an explanation of scope of

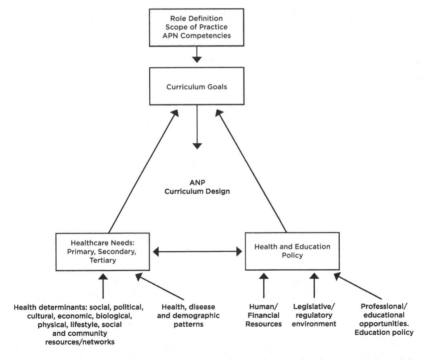

Fig. 4.1 Advanced nursing practice framework for curriculum development (Adapted from Schober and Affara [26], p. 123)

practice and Sect. 4.4 for a discussion of competency statements and core competencies).

A literature review conducted by Schober [25] revealed that various publications are accessed when educational institutions design curricula for ANP with a dominant use of literature originating in the United States. Countries using these resources are then in a position to adapt and modify these aids to fit country context and higher education/healthcare culture. Guidelines, recommendations, and educational frameworks appear to be based mainly on informed and collective academic thinking rather than substantive evidence. No rationale was found in the literature demonstrating outcomes that a specific curriculum was sounder than another for ANP education. Guidelines commonly utilized worldwide appear to be based on advice and/or publications from reputable organizations and sources with an increasingly diverse international representation.

4.3.2   Curriculum Design: Content Distribution

Design and content of a curriculum should be sensitive to the level of advanced practice implicit within the described scope of practice and expected competencies of the program graduates. Identifying fundamental core components at the national level promotes consistency for ANP education within the country across all settings where APNs are envisioned to practice. Figure 4.2 illustrates categories to take into account for the development of a comprehensive and context-sensitive curriculum.

The theory core focuses on the theoretical basis for advanced practice. The clinical core focuses on fundamental clinical modules/courses including in-depth clinical experience in the field. A third category of specialty courses can be tailored to

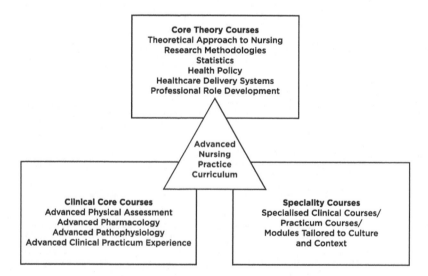

Fig. 4.2   Advanced practice curriculum: course/module distribution [1]

country context or specialty practice (e.g., epidemiology, infectious disease, informatics, mental health, oncology, community health). Adapting ANP education to healthcare needs of the country is imperative. In surveying 14 programs in Australia and New Zealand courses varied but study of pharmacology, research and advanced assessment were common to all [11]. The author acknowledges there is a variety of models and frameworks for ANP education. It must be emphasized that a variety of resources should be reviewed in the developmental process to ensure a context-sensitive approach.

4.4 Program Planning

The international growth of ANP is characterized by diverse requirements for educational preparation as well as the length of requisite study. Programs may consist of select updating modules/courses intended to refine the skills of the generalist nurse to restrictive requirements to qualify for a full academic program. A program manager that has an understanding of the potential scope of practice for APN roles, criteria for student selection, and recruitment of qualified teaching expertise is key to program planning. The following sections discuss student criteria, identification of qualified faculty/teaching staff, teaching strategies, and selection of sites for clinical experience.

4.4.1 Student Criteria

Student criteria for ANP educational preparation vary by country and are based on the level or status of generalist/basic nursing education available. Various studies ([17], [24]) have reported on some of these differences that in turn influence criteria for selecting students. To become an APN, first of all, requires preparation as a generalist nurse. Additional criteria include length of experience as a nurse and experience in a chosen specialty. With the trend toward master's level education and beyond, there is often a requirement to have acquired a bachelor's degree plus clinical experience for entrance into an ANP program. The academic/teaching institution or country standards sets the specific admission criteria.

4.4.1.1 Flexible Criteria Adapted to Context
In the early stages of introducing ANP, it is essential to take into account flexible educational options based on country circumstances. Flexibility in planning and diverse educational pathways allows for continual review, evaluation, and adaptation of APN requirements as ANP and resources evolve. As an initiative is launched, there may be nurses who have worked in APN-like positions without graduate level qualifications but who have acquired competence through appropriate experience and approved diploma or post-basic nursing courses. Country context and healthcare situations will dictate an approach to consider these circumstances. For example, a qualified nurse might be asked to present a portfolio of experiences and be

asked to take specified modules/courses to bridge the gap in order to achieve the equivalence of a master's level qualification. Such a strategy acknowledges the presence of existing nursing capacity while also satisfying education and regulatory authorities.

Nurses are essential to provision of healthcare services in sub-Saharan Africa, but few publications were found regarding ANP in this context. In a qualitative study of ten nurses in Kenya [9], all study participants reported that they were engaged in the delivery of expert-evidenced-based care; however, only two interviewed reported practicing at a level of autonomy similar to that described in the international literature and ICN [14] definition of ANP.

Interestingly, study findings revealed that nurses practicing with the greatest autonomy were generally those with the lowest educational qualifications. Highly qualified nurses tended to choose management and education career paths and saw little opportunity for advancement in a clinical or clinical-academic career. As a result, study findings implied that with no obvious incentive to undertake nursing master's degree participants looked at other options. Lack of a clinical career pathway, scarce access to education opportunities, minimal basic nursing qualifications, and an unsupportive infrastructure present a challenging situation. These issues suggest that flexibility is needed to bridge the education gaps while also attracting young nurses to consider advanced clinical practice.

4.4.1.2 Self-selection

It is common practice in some countries for students to independently select their options for ANP education. In the case of self-selection, a potential student applies to the program and is ultimately accountable and responsible for seeking funding for their education. Academic institutions at times provide assistance to explore options for financial support, but usually the educational institutions themselves do not directly fund fees for study. The United States is an example of a predominantly self-selection application process.

4.4.1.3 External/Institutional Selection

The funding and support within a county can influence the selection of and thus composite of ANP students. When program development falls under the authority of governmental agencies, the selection of students may be coordinated with academic institutions. Supervisors or managers who are familiar with the nurses' work in general practice and/or specialty identify and propose student candidates. Singapore provides an illustration of such a system where the Ministry of Health (MOH) has been pivotal to the feasibility and sustainability of ANP education [25]. An employer (hospital, polyclinic, or healthcare institution) identifies a potential candidate from their current nursing staff. Once selected, the nurse must progress through the university system for graduate student application. Following acceptance and enrollment in the program university fees are funded by the MOH. The employing institution pays a full salary during the time the nurse is an APN student. The nurse applicant agrees to a bonding period with the employer following graduation [25].

4.4.2 Qualified Faculty, Educators, and Teaching Staff

In the beginning stages of an ANP initiative, it is important to explore and remain flexible in the process of identifying professionals qualified to provide expertise to educate nurses for the APN roles. First of all, it is vital that educators, staff, instructors, mentors, and preceptors have an understanding of the scope of practice and competencies for which they are providing education and preparation.

4.4.2.1 Collaborative/Complimentary Educators and Teaching Staff

Environments that lack role models and institutions lacking qualified educators to carry out this role may have to utilize expertise from countries with ANP experience to fill in the gaps, while national educators acquire the necessary competence. Collaborative partnerships with countries or institutions with established success for role development, use of well-informed consultants, and access to a growing body of resources can promote progression to self-sufficiency and sustainability for newly emerging programs. Outside expertise can be considered until a critical mass of national educators are in place.

4.4.2.2 Nursing, Medicine, Other Healthcare Professionals

Internationally there is a widespread concern about the ability to introduce and sustain new ANP programs given the scarcity of qualified educators and staff. Recommendations for suitable teaching staff advise that educators should have a "strong theoretical and practice base in the field in which they teach" (AACN [1], p. 4). Even countries with a successful history of ANP educational programs are facing what some consider human resource crises. In addition, institutions that have educators or staff prepared at the graduate level may not have the knowledge base or the desired level of clinical expertise to teach to the ANP level.

As programs emerge and stabilize their plans and curriculum, healthcare professionals from medicine, nursing, and pharmacy with identified expertise linked to specific modules/courses may be integrated into the teaching profile of the institution to assist in providing learning experiences for APN students. This approach requires assessment and evaluation periodically to determine if teaching strategies are meeting program objectives. In the interim processes for educator/staff enhancement and recruitment are critical for long-term planning and sustainability.

4.5 Teaching Methods

Educators face a complex environment where human and financial resources are scarce and demands are increasing for advanced nursing and multidisciplinary education. The World Health Organization (WHO) has provided guidance for developing relevant education and scaling up the quality of education for healthcare professionals [30]. Taking note of country differences, the WHO document suggests that strategies can vary widely as long as the needs of the country, institution, and learner are taken into consideration. Options or a combination thereof include ad hoc learning situations, class room based teaching, real-life clinical sites, face-to-face interaction, Internet or televideo formats, simulation techniques, and distance learning. Sections 4.5.1 and 4.5.2 discuss e-learning and simulation strategies. It is acknowledged that educators have experience and exposure to other more classic and traditional teaching methods.

4.5.1 Simulation and e-Learning

In the era of technological advancement, e-learning and simulation methods have been increasingly introduced in the educational programs of healthcare professionals including APNs. In informal discussions with educators worldwide, an opinion emerges that these options, while providing exciting new promise for education, should be integrated but not replace all aspects of education and clinical practicum that form the basis for ANP preparation.

4.5.1.1 Simulation

Simulation activities are useful for practicing procedures and techniques that otherwise are not done for practical or ethical reasons. Simulation options are activities using simulation aides to replicate clinical scenarios and can include high and medium fidelity manikins, standardized patients, role-play, computer-based critical thinking simulation, and skill stations. These techniques require experienced staff, space, high-tech equipment, and extensive financial resources. When used, there is evidence that students acquire skills and accelerated learning in a less threatening environment [30].

In a study that looked at the use of simulation as a substitute for traditional clinical experience for undergraduate students, outcomes were similar under the right circumstances to those for traditional clinical teaching [13]. The conclusion from this study was that up to 50 % simulation could be effectively substituted for traditional clinical experience in all core courses in various programs across geographic areas in urban and rural settings. The appropriate circumstances for use of simulation include adequately trained educators, adequate numbers of faculty, dedicated simulation labs, meaningful debriefing, and the funding to sustain this educationalist option.

4.5.1.2 e-Learning

e-Learning (electronic learning) is a combination of content and instructional methods delivered via computers to facilitate a building of knowledge and skills. It assists acquisition and comprehension of knowledge by both offline and online interactive technologies. There are a variety of technologies utilized in e-learning, i.e., Internet, intranets, videos, interactive TV, and CD-ROM. There are several approaches to e-learning including: online learning or web-based instruction, computer-assisted instruction, and virtual classrooms [15].

The use of online education for ANP is dependent on well-structured, interactive, and substantive programs. From specific online modules to complete online ANP programs to Internet access for evidence-based practice cases and study, the age of technology influences education. Desktop computers to hand held devices have made information easily available in many countries. Educators are challenged to continually assess and evaluate the changing learning needs of APN students as newly developing teaching strategies are integrated into curricula. Increasingly students are asked to learn how to locate information efficiently on the Internet, as well as evaluate the validity and relevance of the information. Strategies that teach students' skills in using Internet support are critical in an age of evidence-based practice.

In some countries, complete online modules or courses are offered. A study conducted by Dalhem and Saleh [6] concluded that e-learning, when combined with more traditional methods, had positive outcomes. Duke University in the United States provides one example of this option. In their master's degree (MSN) for ANP, core courses are offered online at least one semester per year. All majors in the MSN program are taught as distance-based or online. While most of the content in a distance-based program is delivered via distance technology, the curriculum includes on-campus intensive sessions that are delivered in a face-to-face, simulation, or hands on format [8].

4.5.2 Clinical Practicum

Clinical on-site student experiences provide opportunities for the student to develop expertise in direct advanced clinical care to individuals, families, or communities. Experiences for clinical learning are significant components of ANP education. Identifying and providing qualified supervision at appropriate clinical sites for the APN students poises challenges for both established and emerging programs. In early phases of program planning, there is a tendency to schedule clinical experiences that are mainly observational. Promoting international visiting to observe practice in countries that have successful and visible APN roles is helpful to gain real-life knowledge of role potential. However, restricting student clinical exposure to observation only does not allow the student to develop the competence expected of a nurse in the APN role.

In addition, in initial phases of ANP education, there may be a reliance on physicians to teach and supervise clinical course/module components and for qualified nursing educators to teach theoretical components that relate to role acquisition and a theoretical approach to nursing. Over time a blending of these approaches leads to interdisciplinary teaching. As a program matures, there will be options for qualified nursing educators/staff to teach most theoretical program components and for APNs to supervise clinical practicum, acting as role models and preceptors. As preceptors and mentors experienced in the role, APNs provide insight for the direction of attaining the knowledge base and skills essential for entry level ANP.

In planning classroom-based courses that prepare for clinical practicum thought should be given to the adequacy of physical space in relation to number of students and accommodation of teaching methods. Adequate space will be needed for demonstration models, clinical simulation experiences, and surrogate patient models when included as teaching strategies. In an era of high-tech teaching methods, it is most advantageous when preparing student clinical learning experiences to provide students access to audiovisual aids, information technology, and Internet access. The opportunity to access resources to expand their technological skills as needed should be considered. The author acknowledges that where resources are limited the resourcefulness of educators will be challenged in providing quality clinical experiences.

4.5.2.1 Preceptors and Mentors: Developing APN Competence

Clinical practice facilitated by a preceptor or a mentor provides APN students real-life experiences to practice clinical skills such as history taking, performance of physical assessments, practice under supervision of diagnostic and care management plans. Management within the clinical setting can include management of acute and chronic illness, health promotion interventions, and referrals to other resources and healthcare professionals. Students entering a specialty clinical practicum are scheduled based on their experience, specialty interest, and available preceptors/mentors. Preceptorship can be identified as:

> a formal one-to-one relationship of pre-determined length, between an experienced [preceptor] and a novice [preceptee] designed to assist the novice in successfully adjusting to a new role...domain or setting (CNA [4], p. 13).

At the start, physicians with expertise in the field or specialty can be called upon to function as preceptors or mentors with guidance from the nursing program manager. Physician preceptors/mentors may be unaccustomed to educating nurses to an advanced level or being evaluated on their performance as a preceptor. Approaching these situations diplomatically is always wise. Provision of a preceptor manual or handbook with guidelines [19, 29] plus periodic meetings with the preceptors can provide helpful direction for teaching, supervising, and evaluating students. It is crucial that preceptors and mentors recognize that the essence of ANP education differs from that provided for the generalist nurse and that it overlaps with but differs from medical practice. In clinical sites, senior or experienced nurses can add to clinical experiences in initial stages. Over time, with an increase of qualified educators and staff plus a presence of APNs, reliance on physicians as preceptors and senior staff nurses as clinical advisors will likely decrease.

4.5.2.2 Clinical Sites

Achieving identified clinical learning objectives necessitates introduction to a variety of healthcare practitioners and clinical sites. Clinical experiences should be varied to ensure that the students meet educational objectives. Sites should be assessed for appropriateness and evaluated periodically for quality of learning and to make sure sites are not being overloaded with a disproportionate number of students [20]. The following issues can offer difficulty in identifying sites for clinical experiences [7]. Program managers alert to these challenges can in turn develop anticipatory strategies for coordination and planning. Potential problems include:

- Limited suitable clinical sites
- Competition for clinical sites with other healthcare students
- Diverse educational objectives for rural, remote, and urban settings
- Limited understanding of expected ANP competencies
- Inadequate communication of projected clinical learning outcomes
- Uncertain and uneven quality of supervision, precepting, and mentoring

(Doucette [7])

Experience, extensive site visits, and observations by the author are consistent with these concerns. One approach to encourage positive clinical experience is to develop written agreements that clarify expectations for the student experience and responsibilities for the sites providing the experiences.

Conclusion

To promote advanced practice nurses as a credible and acceptable addition to the healthcare workforce, high-quality educational programs are essential. This chapter discusses principles that form the foundation for education consistent with a defined scope of practice and competencies for advanced nursing practice. A curriculum framework is suggested along with recommendations for selecting clinical experience sites and identifying appropriate preceptors and mentors for advanced clinical practicums. Emphasis is placed on role preparation that is reflective of the population(s) needing healthcare services.

References

1. American Association of Colleges of Nursing (AACN) (1996) The essentials of master's education for advanced practice nursing. AACN. Washington DC
2. American Association of Colleges of Nursing (AACN) (2016) APRN Clinical Training Task Force Brief. Accessed 21 March 2016 from http://www.aacn.nche.edu/leading_initiatives_news/news/2015/aprn-white- paper
3. APRN Joint Dialogue Group Report (2008) Consensus Model for APRN regulation: Licensure, accreditation, certification & education. Accessed 17 Mar 2016 from https://www.ncsbn.org/Consensus_Model_for_APRN_Regulation_July_2008.pdf
4. Canadian Nurses Association (CNA) (2004) Achieving excellence in professional practice: a guide to preceptorship and mentorship. CNA. Ottawa
5. Criteria for evaluation of nurse practitioner programs (2012) 4th edn. National Organization of Nurse Practitioner Faculties, Washington DC
6. Dalhem WA, Saleh N (2014) The impact of eLearning on nurses' professional knowledge and practice in HMC [Hamad Medical Corporation, Qatar]. Can J Nurs Informatics Volume 9
7. Doucette S, Duff E, Sangster-Gormley E (2005) Nurse practitioner education in Canada: transforming the future. Presented at the National Organization of Nurse Practitioner Faculties annual conference. Accessed 18 Mar 2016 from http://international.aanp.org/Education/Resources
8. Duke University School of Nursing (2016) Master of Science in Nursing Curriculum. Accessed 19 Mar 2016 from https://nursing.duke.edu/academics/programs/msn/master-science-nursing
9. East LA, Arudo J, Loefler M, Evans CM (2014) Exploring the potential for advanced nursing practice role development in Kenya: a qualitative study. BMC Nurs 13:33
10. Gagan MJ, Berg J, Root S (2002) Nurse practitioner curriculum for the 21st century: a model for evaluation and revision. J Nurs Educ 41(5):2002–2006

11. Gardner G, Carryer J, Dunn S, Gardner A (2004) Nurse practitioner standards project: Report to Australian Nursing Council. Australian Nursing Council.
12. Hamric AB (2014) A definition of advanced practice nursing. In: Hamric AB, Hanson CA, Tracy MF, O'Grady ET (eds) Advanced nursing practice: an integrative approach, 5th edn. St. Louis, Elsevier Saunders, pp 67–132
13. Hayden J, Smiley R, Alexander M, Kardon-Edgren S, Jeffries P (2014) The NCSBN National Simulation Study. National Council State Boards of Nursing, Author, Accessed 21 Mar 2016 from https://www.ncsbn.org/685.htm
14. International Council of Nurses (ICN) (2008) The scope of practice, standards and competencies of the advanced practice nurse. ICN Regulation Series, Geneva
15. Kala S, Isaramalai S, Pohthong A (2010) Electronic learning and constructivism: a model for nursing education. Nurs Educ Today 30(1):61–66
16. Kaasalainen R, Martin-Misener R, Kilpatrick K, Harbman P, Bryant-Lukosius D, Donald F, Carter N (2010) A historical overview of the development of advanced practice nursing roles in Canada. Can J Nurs Leadership 23(Special Issue):35–60
17. Ketefian S, Redman RW, Hanucharurnkul S, Masterson A, Neves EP (2001) The development of advanced practice roles: Implications in the international nursing community. INR 48(3):152–163
18. Martin-Misener R, Bryant-Lukosius D, Harbman P, Donald F, Kaasalainen S, Carter N, Kilpatrick K, DiCenso A (2010) Education of advanced practice nurses in Canada. Can J Nurs Leadersh 23(Special Issue):61–84
19. National Organization of Nurse Practitioner Faculties (NONPF) (2016) Partners in nurse practitioner education: a preceptor manual for nurse practitioner programs, faculty, preceptors and students, 2nd edn. NONPF, Washington DC
20. National Organization of Nurse Practitioner Faculties National Task Force on Quality Nurse Practitioner Education (NTF) (2012), NONPF, Washington DC
21. Nursing Council of New Zealand (NCNZ) (2002) The nurse practitioner: responding to health needs. Author: NCNZ
22. Nursing Council of New Zealand (NCNZ) (2014) Nurse practitioner scope of practice: guidelines for applicants. Responding to health needs. Author: NCNZ
23. Pilane CN, Ncube P, Seitio OS (Undated) Ensuring quality in affiliated health Training institutions: Advanced diploma programmes in Botswana. Accessed 18 Mar 2016 from http://international.aanp.org/Education/Resources, RCN, London
24. Pulcini J, Jelic M, Gul R, Loke AY (2010) An international survey on advanced practice nursing education, practice and regulation. J Nurs Scholarsh 42(1):31–39
25. Schober M (2013) Factors influencing the development of advanced practice nursing in Singapore. Doctoral thesis, Sheffield Hallam University, Sheffield Hallam University archives. Accessed 17 Feb 2016 from http://shura.shu.ac.uk/7799/
26. Schober M, Affara F (2006) Advanced nursing practice. Blackwell Publishing, Oxford
27. Seitio OS (2000) The family nurse practitioner in Botswana: issues and challenges. Presentation at the 8th International Nurse Practitioner Conference. San Diego
28. Towers J (2005) After forty years. J Am Acad Nurse Pract 17(1):9–13
29. University of Colorado Colorado Springs (UCCS) (2015) Nurse practitioner site visitor handbook. Colorado Springs: Author. Accessed 19 Mar 2016 from http://www.uccs.edu/Documents/bethel/Handbooks/GRAD_NSG/NP_PracticumPreceptorHandbook-20150115.pdf
30. World Health Organization (WHO) (2013) Transforming and scaling up health professional education and training. WHO, Geneva
31. World Health Organization-Western Pacific Region (WHO-WPRO) (2001) Mid-level and nurse practitioners in the Pacific: models and issues. WHO-WPRO, Manila

Role and Practice Development

5

Abstract

The introduction of advanced nursing practice entails a process that includes consideration of what models, frameworks, or prototypes are suitable for use in the healthcare environment. Assessment of the rationale for interest in these new nursing roles and/or the need for advanced nursing practice services is a starting point to guide development. Evaluation of the institutional and healthcare milieu such as conducting an environmental scan and/or SWOT analysis will bring attention and focus to the receptivity for integrating this concept. Committed advocates supportive of advanced practice nursing roles are vital in order to face the challenges that affect not only healthcare systems but also all healthcare professionals employed in provision of services and the populations receiving the services. This chapter offers a framework to use to assess the environment in order to progress through developmental stages. Topics relevant to institutional planning, inclusion of advanced practice nursing roles in diverse practice settings, relationships with other healthcare professionals and service users are discussed. Strategies to support the advanced practice nurse and ethics specific to advanced nursing practice conclude the chapter.

Keywords

SWOT analysis • Environmental scan • Role support • Ethics • Integration strategies • Developmental framework

The introduction of advanced nursing practice (ANP) entails a process that includes consideration of what models, frameworks, or prototypes are suitable for use in the healthcare environment. Assessment of the rationale for interest in these new nursing roles and/or the need for ANP services is a starting point that guides development. Evaluation of the institutional and healthcare milieu such as conducting an environmental scan will bring attention and focus to the receptivity for integrating this concept. Committed advocates supportive of advanced practice nursing (APN) roles are vital in order to face the challenges that affect not only healthcare systems

© Springer International Publishing Switzerland 2016
M. Schober, *Introduction to Advanced Nursing Practice*,
DOI 10.1007/978-3-319-32204-9_5

but also all healthcare professionals employed in provision of services and the populations receiving the services. This chapter offers a framework and ideas to assess the environment in order to progress through developmental stages. Topics relevant to institutional planning, inclusion of APN roles in diverse practice settings, relationships with other healthcare professionals and service users are discussed. Strategies to support the APN and ethics specific to ANP conclude the chapter.

5.1   Introducing the Role and Function

Even though there is extensive literature to support the value of ANP, a distinct implementation process suitable for all countries and various settings within a country is unclear. A review of available publications indicates that most available studies and narratives originate in more developed countries such as Australia, Canada, New Zealand, countries of the UK, the Netherlands, Ireland, Singapore, Switzerland, and the USA [9–11, 23, 24, 27]. It is uncertain what components are universally applicable beyond these country contexts. Chapter Two includes a comprehensive global overview of country experiences, and additional country references can be found throughout this publication. Accounts with personalized details of other country experiences, successes, and challenges can be helpful in deciding how to proceed.

In the process of launching an ANP initiative, multiple stakeholders and decision makers including the public have the capability to facilitate or impede development. Key stakeholders may include ministries of health, additional national health agencies, consumer representatives, hospital administrators, academic institutions, professional associations, medical directors, educators, labor, healthcare workforce planners, and nursing leaders. Crucial decisions may be made by persons in positions of authority that have a limited understanding of the issues that are important to promoting ANP as a professional able to provide healthcare services.

5.1.1   The PEPPA Framework

In order to facilitate favorable development, implementation, and evaluation of APN roles, Canadian researchers [3] developed the PEPPA (participatory, evidence-based, patient-focused process for advanced practice nursing) Framework. Steps of the framework take into consideration the complexity of healthcare systems in implementing a new role into an existing healthcare system. Based on principles of participatory action research, the PEPPA Framework (Fig. 5.1) for planning and implementation is intended to establish an atmosphere supportive of ANP.

The PEPPA Framework involves a nine-step process. Steps 1–6 concentrate on setting up role structures. Step 7 looks at role processes and beginning implementation and introduction of the APN roles. Steps 8 and 9 seek to accomplish short and long term evaluations of the APN role and model of care with an aim to assess progress and sustainability of agreed-to target aims and outcomes. The following is an interpretative synopsis of the steps in Fig. 5.1.

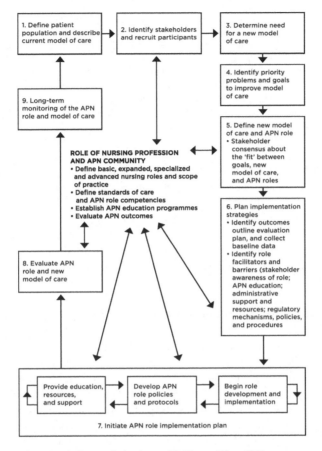

Fig. 5.1 PEPPA framework (Bryant-Lukosius and DiCenso [3], p. 532)

5.1.1.1 PEPPA Framework Steps

Step 1 – Identify the target patient population and establish limits relative to the current model of care.

Step 2 – Key stakeholders and decision makers (including populations and their families) representing the current model of care are invited to contribute input to the discussion of a new model of care that includes the APN role.

Step 3 – Determine the strengths and weakness of the current model of care.

Step 4 – Identify priorities for unmet healthcare concerns with an aim to improve healthcare outcomes.

Step 5 – Define the model of care and healthcare strategies including numbers and mix of healthcare providers. At this time, participants in the process gain an understanding of ANP and various options for APN roles. If the decision is taken to include APNs, a job description and scope of practice is developed that is fit for purpose for the healthcare model.

Step 6 – Strategic implementation planning is done during this step to verify the readiness of the healthcare setting for ANP. This step includes identification of obstacles and facilitators that could influence implementation. Establishing timelines and goals are a critical aspect.

Step 7 – The plan developed in Step 6 for APN implementation is initiated in this step. Full implementation is a continuous process that includes methods to scrutinize various aspects of changes in the approach to provision of healthcare services along with the status of APN role implementation.

Step 8 – Outcomes specific to the identified changes in the model of care are evaluated with a view to identify any needs for APN role development or further role enhancement.

Step 9 – Long term, periodic, and continuous monitoring are emphasized in this step to assess if the model of care integrating APN role continues to be relevant and sustainable.

(Bryant-Lukosius and DiCenso [3])

The PEPPA framework not only provides a comprehensive and practical guide to approaching the inclusion of ANP in provision of healthcare services but also demonstrates the complexity and dynamics of considering such an initiative. Although it may seem overwhelming at first glance, the framework can be used as a flexible guide when deciding how to tailor ANP services for a specific healthcare setting and/or targeted population. The framework has been used in 16 countries with detailed documentation of utilization of the framework in Switzerland [4].

5.1.2   Environmental Scanning and SWOT Analysis

In anticipation of introducing APN roles or refining existing roles assessing the context where these changes will take place can contribute to purposeful planning. Environmental scanning and SWOT (strengths, weaknesses, opportunities, threats) analysis are comprehensive and strategic tools that can be used to establish the level of understanding needed for a successful plan. An environmental scan assists in assessing internal needs and the external environment. Inclusion of the SWOT analysis assists in confirming or disproving widespread perceptions [6, 7]. Although each of these tools can be used independently, using these tools together promotes the collection of information to assist in determining the readiness of a country, institution, or agency for the introduction of ANP.

The environmental scan collects information and data to gain an understanding of the situation. The SWOT analysis categorizes the information as to strengths, weaknesses, opportunities, and threats present in the system. Strengths are internal factors helpful to achieving desired goals; weaknesses are internal factors that may block achievement of objectives; opportunities are external factors that could be beneficial in achieving goals; and threats are external factors that may block achievement of objectives. A completed SWOT matrix can be used to identify strategies to maximize strengths, defeat threats, overcome weaknesses, and take advantage of opportunities in order to set priorities for actions (see Appendices 5.1 and 5.2 at the end of this chapter for a SWOT analysis matrix template and a SWOT analysis illustration).

Conducting an environmental scan along with a SWOT analysis identifies gaps that need to be addressed, thus contributing to development of strategies to close these gaps in order to proceed forward [7]. Information and trends discovered during the environmental scan can provide a basis for a SWOT analysis finding. For example, if the environmental scan predicts a shortage of funding for APN, this can be viewed as a threat to an ANP initiative. A prediction of a physician shortage in primary healthcare can be seen as an opportunity to consider the introduction of ANP. For more detailed guidance on doing an environmental scan that focuses on doing a stakeholder analysis access see http://www.who.int/workforcealliance/knowledge/toolkit/33.pdf, for Part 2 of a World Health Organization's "Policy Toolkit for Strengthening Health Sector Reform."

5.2 Interconnectedness

The inclusion of ANP and APN roles does not occur in isolation. Numerous questions arise as the roles evolve and APNs are required to relate to other nurses, healthcare professionals, organizations/healthcare systems, regulatory systems, and the public. Strategies to facilitate an effective integration of the APN when connecting with various healthcare entities and healthcare professionals are suggested in Sects. 5.2.1, 5.2.2, and 5.2.3.

5.2.1 Between and Within Institutional Environments

Integrating ANP into the healthcare workforce of established institutions will likely change the dynamic of the delivery of healthcare services. Persons in various positions of authority can facilitate or impede such changes. Administrators and managers need to identify what services the APN is expected to offer and how the delivery of these services connects with the healthcare structure. In the face of healthcare reform and rising healthcare costs, healthcare planners will be called upon to propose the cost-effectiveness and value of an additional healthcare professional. A clear explanation and evidence of the beneficial aspects of ANP will strengthen any proposal that aims to integrate the APN roles. Ideally, APNs should promote the value of their practice and thus collaborate with healthcare administrators who are in a position to orchestrate a welcoming institutional environment.

The following question can provide focus when considering an organizational workforce approach:

> *If you were in a position with full authority to create a healthcare model for an institution that included APNs what would it look like?*

At a medical center in the United States, the director of advanced practice professionals responded to that question, sought the input of others, and organized a subcommittee of APNs (nurse practitioners and clinical nurse specialists) in order to come up with a model that could to be implemented in the organization. Discussions led to the creation of a patient-centered, collaborative-care approach intended to decrease hospital readmissions, costs of care, and improve patient outcomes. Outcomes of the model demonstrated that when healthcare disciplines work collaboratively and APNs are given responsibilities that allow them to use their administrative and clinical expertise, there are benefits for patients, physicians, and the organization. The model, which originally focused on heart failure patients, was implemented in January 2012. Over a 12-month period, 30-day readmission rates dropped from 26 to 8 %. Healthcare costs for the identified group of patients receiving care via the new model decreased significantly during 30 days after discharge.

In this model of care by a multidisciplinary team, the APN identified heart failure patients who qualified to be admitted per program criteria, met the patient and family, introduced the APN role, and provided basic patient education in the hospital. In addition, the APN and family scheduled post-discharge follow up for more intensive education sessions. Any necessary follow up with a physician was scheduled as needed. The APN developed a management plan with the physician, ensured all diagnostic tests and reports were completed, assessed if the patient's condition was stable before hospital discharge, and implemented the discharge plan. After discharge, the APN contacted the patient by phone within 24–48 h. During the first follow up visit, the APN performed a full physical assessment and a full educational session along with a family member or support person. The education session included review of diet, daily weights, and a medication management tool. Improved outcomes with this model led to APN care being added to more of the medical center's services including cardiology, chronic care management, oncology, and genetics. In addition, the model's success influenced initiation of APN healthcare service delivery beyond the hospital to community services [19, 28].

5.2.1.1 Strategies for Integrating APN Roles Within Organizational/ Institutional Systems

The following are proposed strategies to consider when preparing to integrate APNs into healthcare systems and institutional settings:

- Develop a clear role definition, scope of practice, and the position of the APN based on the setting where the APN will practice
- Include key decision makers and stakeholders in discussions on the value of ANP to institution services
- Provide outcomes studies and evidence supportive of ANP
- Develop a plan for healthcare workforce planning and skill mix
- Discuss standards, education needs, and regulatory issues
- Consider a framework for strategic planning that includes follow up and evaluation of ANP services
- Make available choices for funding and resources for creating positions, education, and support for competence maintenance

5.2.2 Among Other Settings

In a survey of 32 countries, Pulcini et al. [20] found that over 70 % of roles identified as ANP were in hospital based or institutional settings. However, there appears to be a growing presence in out-of-hospital environments. These settings include primary care/primary healthcare, community, acute/emergency care, and APN-led clinics.

Although the settings are diverse, the key to integration of APNs in these sites, as in hospital/institutional settings, is also familiarity with the role and scope of practice as it relates to the healthcare infrastructure and locale. Systematic patient-focused planning to guide role development along with identification of funding for positions is essential along with support within the organizational structure that allocates a place for new positions. Identifying and integrating the APN in the system is ultimately necessary for effective functioning of the system. The complexities and diversity of various systems of care, even within the same country, can be daunting. Discussions are not always positive and can be argumentative when discussing changes that involve professional boundaries.

De Geest et al. [9] recommend a conceptual framework to analyze the introduction of APN roles through five drivers. The identified drivers are: (1) the healthcare needs of the population, (2) education, (3) workforce, (4) practice patterns, and (5) legal and health policy framework (p. 626). Similarly, Blair and Jansen [29] suggest that an assessment and understanding of the setting and healthcare environment or culture is a necessity when preparing to introduce the APN role. An awareness of these multifaceted dimensions is likely to identify if the setting is able to implement the changes needed for the APN to practice effectively (see also Sect. 5.1.1 on environmental scanning and SWOT analysis).

5.2.3 Between Other Healthcare Professionals

In the process of role acquisition and implementation, boundaries for APN roles based on basic nursing principles are in a state of flux. APNs usually take on some skills and critical thinking associated with care management that has traditionally been associated with medicine. This raises questions about the APNs' professional scope of practice as nurses. Schober and Affara [25] posed the question "When is a nurse no longer a nurse?" (p. 60). Nurses in advanced roles express uncertainty about their place in the healthcare settings in which they practice and report adverse working relationships with other nurses [12, 24]. In a study conducted in the Netherlands [22], physicians viewed the APN as demonstrating a positive effect on the identity of nurses but the nurses themselves did not share this view reporting that they were conflicted about role expectations. APNs in this study portrayed conflict about expectations for the role. From one perspective the APN is expected to be a nurse while there are also expectations of the role that is more closely aligned with medicine.

5.2.3.1 Relations with Nursing
It can happen that in the process of introducing APN roles to a healthcare setting, other nurses are not necessarily receptive to the idea. In some situations physicians are the advocates for ANP, while nursing colleagues abandon the novice APN, or are reluctant to facilitate advanced practice opportunities for practice. In a study conducted in Singapore [24], the nurses viewed the APNs as not belonging to the nursing culture anymore. In addition, there was a view that APNs no longer practiced nursing but acted like physicians.

Nursing managers, sometimes with limited knowledge of the role, are usually responsible for the implementation of APN services and may be uncertain as to how the role should be implemented [8, 14, 21]. The issue of role ambiguity [12] appears to add to the skepticism exhibited by other nurses expected to work with the APN. Reay et al. [21] address the anticipated facilitative role of nurse managers and recommend that managers: (1) clarify reallocation of tasks, (2) manage altered relations in the healthcare team, and (3) continue to actively manage the healthcare team in evolving circumstances to ease relations between APNs and other nurses. Consistent with the recommendations by Reay et al. [21], the following strategies are proposed to promote more amicable relations between APNs and other nursing staff.

Strategies for Facilitating Relations with Other Nurses

- Clearly define and differentiate the APN role from other nurses in the healthcare setting and healthcare workforce.
- Provide a clear and visible description of the APN and expected scope of practice.
- Identify any areas of concern by nursing staff related to introducing this new nursing role along with actively taking steps to resolve any concerns.
- Facilitate communication between all nurses to develop understanding of their respective positions in the healthcare workforce. e.g., conferences, workshops, meetings that require decisions associated with both roles.

5.2.3.2 Relations with Medical Colleagues

Resolving collegial relationships between two autonomous practitioners such as APNs and doctors with substantial overlap in their scope of practice requires the utmost diplomacy at times. Even though APNs and doctors share certain competencies, the focus of their practice is different. However, turf battles can occur when professionals compete to perform the same tasks. Evidence on the issue of physician support is mixed with respondents in two studies citing medical group opposition on the one hand [20] and limited physician opposition on the other [17]. However, medical dominance and control over healthcare services in many countries indicate this group of healthcare professionals has the ability and authority to impede or support optimal utilization of APNs. Baerlocher and Detsky [1] recommend negotiation that focuses on keeping the publics' rather than the professions' interests in mind. The following strategies are suggested to enhance a positive environment.

Strategies for Facilitating Positive Communication with Medical Colleagues

- Make available a clear role definition and scope of practice for the APN.
- Involve medical practitioners in collaborative efforts such as developing practice guidelines or standards within a healthcare facility.
- Clearly position the APN in the nursing professional group.
- Define the position of the APN within the healthcare workforce including what a person in this position is expected to do.

- Support attendance at conferences or workshops on topics where all healthcare professionals discuss case management.
- Emphasize collaborative management of patient populations.

The path to introducing the APN role for the individual APN, especially in the early stages, is not simple. Experiencing conflict and a sense of isolation is a common experience [24]. Section 5.3 emphasizes the importance of developing support strategies for the APN.

5.3   Role Support for the Advanced Practice Nurse

Introducing a new nursing role and being the first to provide ANP services can be a solitary experience. Acceptance from other professionals can be limited and conditional until the APN is able to demonstrate competence and confidence in the role. The public may be interested and curious but confused, especially when used to seeking care with a physician. Managers may be enthusiastic but unable to provide the professional support the APN seeks. Lack of support can be disheartening, particularly when there is doubt as to the legitimacy of a nurse functioning in a manner associated with medical practice rather than nursing.

Role development for APNs is viewed by Brykczynski [5] as a two-phase process of role acquisition in the educational program and role implementation after program completion. New graduates were found by Sullivan-Bentz et al. [26] to move from feeling overwhelmed to confident in their ability to function. Additional research on acquisition of knowledge and skills proposes that a progression through stages of performance from novice to expert takes place over time [2, 13].

In a study conducted in Singapore, APNs reported that the nurses no longer viewed the APNs as part of the nursing staff and medical consultants were confused and initially resistant to the new function of these nurses [24]. Sullivan-Bentz et al. [26] examined role transition and support requirements for nurse practitioner (NP) graduates in their first year of practice in Canada and found that the healthcare environment was ill prepared to receive the NPs. In addition, professional territoriality, regulatory barriers, and policies limiting their ability to practice to the full scope of practice negatively impacted inclusion of the role. Study finding by Sullivan-Bentz et al. [26] also revealed that staff and professionals might not be aware of the anxiety new NPs face. Development of strategies to prepare for the inclusion of APNs into healthcare settings with identification of how the strategies will be implemented by healthcare professionals and administrators is vital.

5.3.1   Strategies to Support Advanced Practice Nurses

Preparing students for the realities of the work place that include anticipatory guidance for role transition is possible in theory; however, multiple strategies deserve consideration to support the actual real life process of integrating the APN role into various practice settings. Recommended strategies include the following:

- Identify interprofessional mentor/relationships/supervision before the APN begins employment. An identified mentor can function as a role advocate.
- Clarify reporting mechanisms and expectations of the APN.
  - Who does the APN report to? nursing, medicine, or both
  - Evaluation to be done by: nursing, medicine, or both
- Physicians, allied health professionals, administrators, receptionists, and other nurses *all* receive clear descriptions of role and scope of practice.
- Periodic scheduled meetings.
- Peer support groups – formal and informal; internal and external to the healthcare organization.
  - Provide opportunities to exchange experiences and develop problem solving techniques
  - Opportunities and strategies to resolve barriers and obstacles arising
- Professional development/continuing competence maintenance
  - Interprofessional and joint education/learning experiences
- Designate funding for educational conferences, workshops, meetings

Integration of ANP into the healthcare workforce is a process that takes time. Lack of knowledge of what an APN can contribute to healthcare services in a specific practice setting leads new and inexperienced APNs to develop their role based on an interpretation of theory learned in educationalist preparation [24, 26]. The new APN graduate may define aspects of the role differently from management and other healthcare professionals leading to a sense of disillusionment and disappointment by both the APN and the systems in which they work. Identifying methods of support provides encouragement for the APN in transition to a new role and prepares the healthcare environment and the public for the ANP services that will be provided.

5.4   Situational Ethics

The issue of ethical decision making is fundamental to all nursing practice; however, the APN is in a position as a clinical leader to take on a more vital role in identifying moral and ethical dilemmas, creating ethical environments, and promoting social integrity within healthcare systems [16]. It is not within the scope of this chapter to provide an in-depth discussion of ethics and ethical decision making, but to draw attention to the level of ethical decision making manifest in ANP. (The reader is referred to the ICN *Code of Ethics for Nurses* [18] and a discussion by Hamric and Delgado [16] specific to ANP on this topic.)

The capacity for APNs to participate in ethical decisions arises from their clinical expertise and collaborative proficiency. As nursing leaders in advanced practice with clinical insight, APNs identify ethical dilemmas. In their advanced capacity, APNs have the capacity to assess and facilitate the decision-making process. The autonomous responsibilities and independent decision making associated with APN roles modifies the interchange between nurses and physicians when approaching an ethical situation. Disagreements based on differing professional views with dual professional accountability usually occur in connection to patient care management

[15]. An ethical dilemma occurs when responsibilities require that a person confronts alternative actions but cannot carry out all of them. Conflict occurs when varying demands and choices exist, all of which are unpleasant [16].

For example, in the following scenario an APN determines a woman is a victim of domestic violence based on the APN's assessment. The patient denies there is any such problem. The APN is faced with reporting the situation to the appropriate existing supportive services and putting at risk the professional-client relationship, or avoiding any interference in the situation and possibly allowing the abuse to continue. In this case, the APN consults with the medical consultant on duty. The consultant advises the APN to ignore the situation in order to complete the workload for the day. Based on a model for ethical analysis and decision making proposed by Fry and Johnstone [15], questions the APN can consider include:

What is the significance of the conflict to the involved parties?
Nurses, including APNs, often find that to disagree with a doctor is unpleasant and try to avoid confrontation. In many clinical settings the authority of the doctor is accepted without question. If the medical consultant views the APN as agreeable and collaborative their professional relationship remains intact. The APN could privately provide the woman advice, but this could undercut her credibility and the woman's trust in the physician in addition to comprising care for this woman.

What should be done?
By asking this question the APN considers options for resolving the conflict.

It is important to respect collegial relationships; however, the APN has a responsibility to facilitate reasonable and credible care. In this situation the issues and concerns about the case should be discussed openly with the medical consultant and cannot ethically be avoided. There is not always one correct ethical decision but a decision that is based on the values of those involved, known relevant information, and best judgment on what to do.

Hamric and Delgado [16] discuss general themes for APNs to take into account to decrease uncertainty in ethical decision-making. These include clarifying communication problems, resolving interdisciplinary conflict, and balancing multiple commitments. Specific ethical decisions may be unique to the specialty clinical setting in which the APN practices and are heightened with ANP as a consequence of their advanced clinical expertise and presence in interdisciplinary teams. APNs should obtain competence in this area to avoid power struggles, lead effective communication, and facilitate decisions in ethically difficult situations. Acquired competence increases the ability of an APN to resolve ethically demanding situations.

Conclusion
Introducing and promoting ANP within the healthcare workforce is complex involving institutions, diverse healthcare settings, healthcare managers, and other healthcare professionals. The APNs themselves require encouragement as they initiate a new nursing role with advanced capabilities, especially when there

are no role models. Key decisions may be made by influential individuals in positions of authority with diverse levels of understanding as to the function and capabilities of APNs in providing healthcare services. Other nurses and medical professionals are likely to approach the integration of ANP with caution. This chapter identifies key topics to clarify when introducing the role and suggests approaches to issues that could arise. Strategies for providing role support for APNs are offered and ethical decision making specific to ANP is discussed.

5.5   Appendix 5.1. SWOT Analysis Matix Template

	STRENGTHS	WEAKNESSES
INTERNAL FACTORS		
	OPPORTUNITIES	THREATS
EXTERNAL FACTORS		

Appendix 5.1 SWOT Analysis Matix Template

5.6   Appendix 5.2. SWOT Analysis Illustration

	STRENGTHS	WEAKNESSES
INTERNAL FACTORS	• Observable presence of nurses working in APN roles • Confirmed acceptance by the public • Commitment by nursing to develop • Advanced clinical roles • Respected status of nurses • Accessible advanced nursing education • Funding available for education and positions for an APN	• Poor role definition/ Role ambiguity • Multiple titles to define the same role • Variability in standards of educational programs for advanced nursing • No role models for advanced practice • Regulations lag behind actual practice • Policies limiting advanced practice • Resistance by doctors of APN roles
	OPPORTUNITIES	THREATS
EXTERNAL FACTORS	• Increasing educational levels for nursing • Move to university based nursing education • Growing demand of healthcare services for chronic/long term illness • Healthcare reform & governmental desire to improve care • Shortage of doctors • Interest in new models of healthcare provision, e.g. collaborative, multidisciplinary teams	• Identification of new categories of healthcare professionals viewed as a possible threat to APN development, e.g. physician assistants • Medical dominance • Absence of professional development/career pathways • Lack of qualified faculty to prepare APNs • Lack of defined scopes of practice or approved posts/positions for the APN • Inadequate funding for education

Appendix 5.2 SWOT Analysis Illustration

References

1. Baerlocher M, Detsky A (2009) Professional monopolies in medicine. JAMA 301(8):858–860
2. Benner P (1984) From novice to expert: excellence and power in clinical nursing practice. Addison-Wesley, Menlo Park
3. Bryant-Lukosius D, DiCenso A (2004) A framework for the introduction and evaluation of advanced practice nursing roles. J Adv Nurs 48(5):530–540

4. Bryant-Lukosius D, Spichinger E, Martin J, Stoll H, Kellerhals SD, Fleidner M, Grossman F, Henry M, Hermann L, Koller A, Schwendimann R, Ulrich A, Weibel L, Callen SB, De Gesst S (2016) Framework for evaluating the impact of advanced practice nursing roles. J Nurs Scholarsh 48(2):201–209. doi:10.1111/jnu.12199

5. Brykczynski KA (2014) Role development of the advanced practice nurse. In: Hamric AB, Hanson CM, Tracy MF, O'Grady ET (eds) Advanced practice nursing: an integrative approach, 5th edn. Elsevier Saunders, St. Louis, pp 328–358

6. Canadian Nurses Association (CNA) (2011) Board of directors environmental scan. Author: CNA, Ottawa

7. CPS Human Resource Services (2007) Workforce planning toolkit: environmental scan and SWOT analysis. Retrieved 12 Apr 2016 from http://www.cpshr.us/workforceplanning/documents/ToolKitGap-Closing.pdf

8. Currie K, Tolson D, Booth J (2007) Helping or hindering: the role of nurse managers in the transfer of practice development learning. J Nurs Manag 15(6):585–594

9. De Geest S, Moons P, Cailens B, Gut C, Lindpainter L, Spirig R (2008) Introducing advanced practice nurses/nurse practitioners in health care systems: a framework for reflection and analysis. Swiss Med Wkly 138(43-44):621–628

10. Delemaire M, LaFortune G (2010) Nurses in advanced roles: a description and evaluation of experiences in 12 developed countries. OECD Health Working Papers, No. 54, OECD Publishing. doi:10.1787/5kmbrcfms5g7-en

11. DiCenso A, Bryant-Lukosius D, Bourgeault I, Martin-Misener R, Donald F, Abelson J, Kaasalainen S, Kilpatrick K, Kioke S, Carter N, Harbman P (2010) Clinical nurse specialists and nurse practitioners in Canada: a decision support synthesis. Canadian Health Services Research Foundation, Ottawa

12. Donald F, Bryant-Lukosius D, Martin-Misener R, Kaasalainen S, Kilpatrick K, Carter N, Harbman P, Bourgeault I, DiCenso A (2010) Clinical nurse specialists and nurse practitioners: title confusion and lack of role clarity. Can J Nurs Leadership 23(Special Issue):189–210

13. Dreyfus HL, Dreyfeus SE (2009) The relationship of theory and practice in the acquisition of skill. In: Benner P, Tanner CA, Chesla (eds) Expertise in nursing practice: caring, clinical judgment and ethics. 2nd edn. Springer, New York, pp 1–23

14. Fang L, Tung H (2010) Comparison of nurse practitioner job core competency expectations of nurse managers, nurse practitioners, and physicians in Taiwan. JAANP 22:409–416

15. Fry ST, Johnstone MJ (2008) Ethics in nursing practice: a guide to ethical decision making, 3rd edn. Wiley – Blackwell Publishing, Oxford

16. Hamric AB, Delgado SA (2014) Ethical decision making. In: Hamric AB, Hanson CM, Tracy MF, O'Grady ET (eds) Advanced practice nursing: an integrative approach, 5th edn. Elsevier Saunders, St. Louis, pp 328–358

17. Heale R, Rieck Buckley C (2015) An international perspective of advanced practice nurse regulation. Int Nurs Rev 62(3):421–429

18. International Council of Nursing (ICN) (2012) Code of ethics for nurses. Author, Geneva

19. Kutzleb J, Rigolosi R, Fruhschien A, Reilly M, Shaftic AM, Duran D, Flynn D (2015) Nurse practitioner care model: meeting the health care challenges with a collaborative team. Nurs Econ 33(6):297–304

20. Pulcini J, Jelic M, Gul R, Loke AY (2010) An international survey on advanced practice nursing education, practice and regulation. J Nurs Scholarsh 42(1):31–39

21. Reay T, Golden-Biddle K, Germann K (2003) Challenges and leadership strategies for managers of nurse practitioners. J Nurs Manag 11(6):396–403

22. Roodbol P (2005) Willing o'-the-wisps, stumbling runs, toll roads and song lines: study into the structural rearrangement of tasks between nurses and physicians. Summary of a doctoral thesis. Unpublished

23. Sastre-Fullana P, De Pedro-Gomez JE, Bennasar-Veny M, Serrano-Gallardo P, Morales-Ascencio JM (2014) Competency frameworks for advanced practice nursing: a literature review. Int Nurs Rev 61(4):534–542

24. Schober M (2013) Factors influencing the development of advanced practice nursing in Singapore. Doctoral thesis, Sheffield Hallam University, U.K., Sheffield Hallam University archives. Accessed 05 Mar 2016 from http://shura.shu.ac.uk/7799/

25. Schober M, Affara F (2006) Advanced nursing practice. Blackwell Publishing Ltd, Oxford

26. Sullivan-Bentz M, Humbert J, Cragg B, Legault F, Laflamme C, Bailey PH, Doucette S (2010) Supporting primary health care nurse practitioners' transition to practice. Can Fam Physician 56(11):1176–1182

27. Ter Maten-Speksnijder A, Grypdonck M, Pool A, Meurs P, van Staa AL (2013) A literature review of the Dutch debate on the nurse practitioner role: efficiency vs. professional development. Int Nurs Rev 61:44–54

28. Thew J (2016) NP care model drastically lowers heart failure readmissions. HealthLeaders Media, online publication HealthLeadersMedia.com

29. Zwilling JG (2015) Advanced practice nursing within health care settings. In: Blair KA, Jansen MP (eds) Advanced practice nursing: core concepts for professional role development, 5th edn. Springer Publishing Company, New York, pp 57–66

Professional Regulation

6

Abstract

Professional regulation is the legitimate and appropriate means – governmental, professional, private, and individual – whereby order, identity, consistency, and control are brought to the profession. Professional regulation for advanced nursing practice consists of the rules and policies that recognize the advanced practice nurse and officially credentials advanced practice nurses for practice. This chapter describes the significance of having appropriate regulatory mechanisms in place for professional practice to support advanced practice nurses to the full potential of their role within the context of a country's healthcare system and settings. It begins with the International Council of Nurses guidelines for establishing advanced nursing practice professional regulation. Additional regulatory frameworks and models are offered in order to provide examples to consult in the process of formalizing the policies and processes associated with regulation. Topics relevant to advanced nursing practice credentialing including accreditation, certification, licensure, registration, and endorsement are discussed. The chapter concludes with a comprehensive overview of maintaining practice competence.

Keywords

Professional regulation • Legislation • Credentialing • Standards • Competence maintenance

Professional regulation is the legitimate and appropriate means – governmental, professional, private, and individual – whereby order, identity, consistency, and control are brought to the profession. The profession and its members are defined; the scope of practice is determined; standards of education, ethical, and competent practice are set; and systems of accountability are established through these means [14]. Professional regulation for advanced nursing practice (ANP) consists of the rules and policies that recognize the advanced practice nurse (APN) and officially credential APNs for practice [12]. This chapter describes the significance of having appropriate regulatory mechanisms in place for professional practice to support APNs to the full potential of their role within the context of a country's healthcare system and settings. It begins with the ICN guidelines for establishing advanced nursing practice (ANP) professional regulation. Regulatory frameworks and models are offered in order to have examples to consult in the process of formalizing the policies and processes of regulation. Topics relevant to ANP credentialing, including accreditation, certification, licensure, registration, and endorsement are discussed. The chapter concludes with a comprehensive overview of maintaining practice competence.

Legislation and professional regulation ideally should grant a distinct title designation and protection for the APN, justify the role, and award clear authority to carry out a range of activities related to ANP. Through a formally authorized institution or agency, professional regulation has a function to legitimatize the role, protect the public, as well as to monitor individual healthcare professionals practice and behavior. This purpose also serves to hold healthcare providers accountable for their actions in an effort to protect the public and offer safe, quality healthcare service. The organization or agency regulating nursing uses current scope of practice and standards to disseminate policy and regulations. These provide direction and acknowledgement of professional educational preparation and boundaries of practice. ICN has recommended minimal standards for the professional regulation of ANP. These guidelines are as follows:

- Develop and maintain sound credentialing mechanisms that enable the authorized nurse to practice in the advanced role within an established scope of practice
- Establish relevant civil legislation or rules to acknowledge the authorized role, monitor APN competence and protect the public through issuance of guidance, assessment processes and when necessary, fitness to practice procedures and processes
- Periodically revise professional regulatory language to maintain currency with nursing practice and scientific advancement
- Establish title protection through rule making or civil legislation.

(ICN 2008, p. 21 [15])

In the process of developing a professional regulatory model or framework, clarifying the definition of ANP and the APN roles is vital when explaining the concept to external stakeholders such as legislators and healthcare planners Hamric [11]. Identifying core features of APN roles such as entry-level education, certification, licensure, and the focus of practice are key elements in delineating professional regulation and credentials specific to ANP. The next section provides guidelines and framework examples to consider when pursuing regulatory structure.

6.1 Frameworks and Models for Professional Regulation

A well-defined framework is key to achieving consistency and sustainability of the APN role and allows ANP to evolve as a distinct and legitimate part of the healthcare delivery system. Credentialing of APNs is the central function of the regulatory system arising out of this framework. Credentialing is discussed later in this chapter (see Sect. 6.1.1). Factors likely to influence development of a professional regulatory framework include:

- Type and stability of the political system in the country
- Legislative and regulatory traditions of the country
- Regional and international trends that influence regulation
- The level of detail wanted/required in the regulatory system
- The rate of change in educational standards, practice and technology
- Time, human expertise and financial resources needed to enact or revise regulations

Schober and Affara [29]

Dimensions of Regulation are proposed in the Healthcare Professional and Occupational Regulation Toolkit [16]. A recommendation is made that a series of questions to ask can be useful in discussing and developing a professional regulatory structure. The questions include:

- *WHY* or for what purpose is a regulation created?
- *WHAT* is regulated? Targets of the regulatory system could include persons providing service, educational programs preparing the professional and/or institutions.
- *WHO is the authority* that licenses, registers, certifies, approves, or accredits persons, programs, or institutions?
- *WHO carries out* the regulation?
- *HOW* are regulation or credentialing mechanisms *carried out*?
- *HOW are methods and tools used* in the regulatory processes to review and evaluate qualifications? How do you know standards have been met?

Criteria for measuring the extent to which standards have been met include codes of professional conduct, civil service requirements, and disciplinary procedures. Validation tools, such as national examinations, school records, letters of recommendation, portfolios, interviews, institutional self- assessment, visits to facilities, and healthcare records, are other means used to gain evidence of knowledge, performance, and outcomes [16]. For further discussion of performance maintenance refer to Sect. 6.3.

6.1.1 The ICN Credentialing Framework: A Basis for ANP Professional Regulatory Structure

The degree of detail required for components of a professional regulatory model or framework for ANP is country specific. A model (see Table 6.1) based on the ICN Credentialing Framework [13] offers a point of reference to begin to change or reform a professional regulatory structure. The ICN framework proposes the following characteristics:

Table 6.1 Professional regulatory model for advanced nursing practice (Schober and Affara [29], p. 103)

Law	Regulations
Definition of APN	Scope of practice definition
Title protection	Standards and guidelines
	Entry into practice requirements
	Level of education
	Practice
	Assuring competence maintenance
	Professional conduct
Regulatory body	Processes/procedures for certain regulatory activities
Composition	Credentialing
Powers and functions	Providing examinations, reviews, interviews
Appointment and conditions for office	Accreditation of educational programs/institutions
	Renewal, suspension, removal, reinstatement of license
	Hearings/consultations
	Complaint and disciplinary proceedings
Dealing with other jurisdictions	Communication
	Reporting
Resources for conducting affairs (power to raise revenue)	Data collected about credentialee
	Evaluating regulatory effectiveness

In the Law Title protection, APN definition, nature of the agency responsible to regulate the APN along with designated functions, and powers of the agency and its authority to conduct regulatory transactions are given a level of protection provided by the law.

In the Regulations Components more sensitive to modifications in practice, knowledge, and healthcare delivery can be addressed through regulations that include interpretation thus allowing for flexibility to respond to change in healthcare systems, healthcare settings, professional, and alterations within the public domain.

Table 6.1 demonstrates the diversity of factors requiring consideration in developing a professional regulatory model/framework for ANP. Issues that need to be discussed for inclusion in a model or framework include: titling (name and level of protection), scope of practice (level of authority and autonomy), educational requirements, types of credentialing mechanisms, and renewal of credentials and methods for validating/evaluating competence.

6.1.2   SSPP Model (Scope, Standards, Policies, and Procedures)

In the SSPP model, scopes of practice, professional standards, policies, and procedures (SSPP) are linked in a logical manner with one being the foundation stone for another [16]. Figure 6.1 illustrates how professional standards grow out of the definition of a profession's scope of practice. The scope of practice identifies and communicates the health professional's range of activities – roles, functions, responsibilities, activities, accountability, decision-making capacity, and authority.

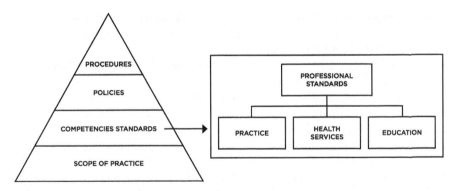

Fig. 6.1 SSPP model (scope, standards, policies, procedures) (Access from https://reprollneplus. org/system/files/resources/03_SSPP%20Model_tc.pdf)

Competencies and standards are derived from a process of linking a situational analysis, task analysis, and scope of practice definitions.

This model provides a comprehensive approach that includes introductory regulatory concepts and principles to guide key stakeholders in development of a professional regulatory framework. Defining a scope of practice for APN roles forms the foundation of the SSPP model. Scopes of practice are essential regulatory means that form the basis of APN practice. Scopes of practice inform standards and competencies, communicate role expectations, and inform curriculum content and practice standards. In addition, the defined scope of practice identifies the function of the APN, differentiates this level of nurse from other categories of nurses and healthcare professionals, and assists in the process of healthcare workforce planning.

Resting on the foundation of an established scope of practice is a defined set of competencies required of the APN for safe and capable practice. The competencies are linked to role, practice, and education. Competence in healthcare is the capacity to deliver a specified healthcare service effectively and safely. Regulators use competencies to ensure healthcare professionals function skillfully within their defined scope of practice. (Refer to Chap. 3 – Nature of Practice for further discussion on developing ANP scopes of practice).

In the SSPP model, the setting of standards includes establishing procedures and policies that provide the basis of professional accountability and autonomy. Standard setting is considered to be a central part of what professional organizations, regulatory bodies, and governmental agencies offer to a professional discipline such as ANP in the process of role development.

6.1.3   National Examples of Models and Frameworks

In order to offer a pragmatic perspective of the regulatory processes for ANP, country specific examples are presented in the following sections (Sects. 6.1.3.1, 6.1.3.2, 6.1.3.3, and 6.1.3.4) to provide descriptions of approaches taken by the selected countries with varied lengths of experience with APN roles.

6.1.3.1 USA National Model. Consensus for Advanced Practice Registered Nurse Regulation: Licensure, Accreditation, Certification and Education

In the United States, until recently, there was no common ground for regulating the field of ANP that includes certified registered nurse anesthetists, certified nurse-midwives, certified nurse practitioners, and clinical nurse specialists. Core issues had been taken up by universities over the years in educating the various APNs. Leaders from professional nursing associations, certifying bodies, and regulators took the lead in 2004 to establish a process that resulted in a consensus statement on credentialing of APNs (APRN [advanced practice registered nurse] is the agreed title in the USA) and ultimately a regulatory model that established a model for education, certification, accreditation, and licensure [12]. The vision was to have one national regulatory scheme that would be beneficial to patients and allow APNs to meet patient needs [22]. The Consensus Model as of May 2016 is endorsed by 48 national nursing organizations. Even though the model is a reality and is coordinated with credentialing stakeholders, differences for credentialing APNs continue to exist across the 50 states. It is speculated that it will take time to fully implement this model [12].

The Consensus Model has wide-ranging impact on licensing boards, accreditation agencies, certification organizations, and educational programs. Some of the significant highlights of the model follow next:

- The Consensus Model defines four APRN roles: certified registered nurse anesthetist (CRNA), certified nurse-midwife (CNM), clinical nurse specialist (CNS), and certified nurse practitioner (CNP). These four roles are given the title of advanced practice registered nurse (APRN).
- Education, certification, and licensure of an individual must be congruent in terms of role and population foci.
- The model calls for all APRNs to be educated in an accredited graduate-level education program in one of the four roles and in at least one of six population foci: family/individual across the lifespan, adult-gerontology, pediatrics, neonatal, women's health/gender-related, or psych/mental health.
- The emphasis for all APRNs is that a significant component of their education and practice focuses on direct clinical care of individuals.
- All APRNs must be educated/prepared to assume responsibility for health promotion as well as assessment, diagnosis, and management of patient concerns, which includes the use and prescription of pharmacologic and nonpharmacologic interventions whether or not an APRN later chooses to gain prescriptive authority.
- All APRNs are required to pass a national certification examination and required to maintain continued competence verified through a recertification process with a national certification agency.
- Advanced practice registered nurses are licensed practitioners expected to practice within standards established or recognized by a licensing body.

Credentialing for APRNs is composed of: licensure, accreditation, certification, and education. The acronym LACE is used to refer to these four components. More extensive details on the Consensus Model can be found on https://www.ncsbn.org/736.htm and http://www.nonpf.org/?page=26

6.1.3.2 New Zealand: Adapting Professional Regulations

The nurse practitioner (NP) was a new scope of nursing practice launched by the Ministry of Health and the Nursing Council of New Zealand in 2001 [19]. Following extensive consultation in 2015, the Nursing Council of New Zealand made an announcement that changes will be made to the nurse practitioner scope of practice and education programs that prepare nurse practitioners to meet future health needs of New Zealanders. These changes are expected to come into effect in 2016. The scope of practice has been broadened and the requirement to restrict nurse practitioners to a specific area of practice has been removed. This model has been safely implemented in Australia and offered guidance in New Zealand. Nurse practitioners, as advanced clinicians, will be expected to self-regulate and practice within their area of competence and experience.

Nurse practitioners in New Zealand have demonstrated safe advanced practice since they were first regulated in 2001. The Nursing Council thinks that the changes will allow greater flexibility for nurse practitioners to meet future healthcare needs of the country. A revised scope of practice provided by the Council also makes the role and contribution of nurse practitioners clearer to employers and the public, and differentiates the nurse practitioner from other advanced registered nurse roles.

As previously indicated, the new scope of practice statement for the nurse practitioner will be introduced in 2016. Nurse practitioner candidates will still have an opportunity to focus on an area of practice but it will not appear on the register or on their practicing certificate. Nurse practitioner candidates will be expected to complete the same or similar papers as registered nurses preparing to prescribe for long-term and common conditions as part of their program. This will broaden their skills and knowledge and create greater consistency in their preparation. It will also prepare them to be able to mentor registered nurses who are learning to prescribe.

The Nursing Council of New Zealand also decided to refocus education programs to prepare nurse practitioners so that they will have more specific program outcomes that include 300 h of protected clinical learning time. It is anticipated that these changes will lead to greater consistency and range in nurse practitioner preparation to hopefully improve readiness for registration upon completion of their education program. Currently the Nursing Council of New Zealand accredits clinical master's programs as the required qualification for nurse practitioners. Over the years these programs have become increasingly diverse as they have sought to meet the needs of newly graduated nurses, nurses in diverse specialties, and nurses who wish to become educators, mangers, and researchers. The Council has decided to accredit specific nurse practitioner programs with consistent outcomes that lead to nurse practitioner registration.

In reviewing current regulations and policies for NPs, the Nursing Council of New Zealand is also investigating:

- The possibility of requiring a year supervision for newly registered NPs
- Developing new competencies that accurately reflect the new scope of practice
- Whether it is necessary to submit a portfolio to demonstrate clinical competence when applying for registration
- Ways to better ensure consistent standards for candidate assessment.

NCNZ [28]

The consultations and reexamination of NP regulations sought by the Nursing Council of New Zealand offers an example of an adaptive approach to adjusting professional regulations following 15 years of experience with the NP role. Over time and with experience, as the concept of ANP matures, professional regulations will require modification.

6.1.3.3 The Scottish Advanced Nursing Practice Framework: A Toolkit Approach

Deliberations in the UK on regulating ANP have been complex, spanning over 20 years. Debates started in the late 1980s and early 1990s as service and strategic interest in advanced nursing roles increased. Despite a great deal of strategic intent and service change, professional regulation across the UK remains unresolved and is now widely regarded as unachievable and unwarranted [2]. The Council for Healthcare Regulatory Excellence [5] in the UK outlined the complexity of professional regulatory issues and made it clear that, in its view, the code of professional conduct [24, 25] encompasses advanced practitioner practice, thus negating any need for additional formal regulation [2]. Indirectly that perspective led to the development of the Advanced Nursing Practice Toolkit [30] under the auspices of the Modernising Nursing Careers report [6]. This began to provide some national conformity and guidance to employers, practitioners, and educators. Subsequently and following the release in 2009 of the NHS Scotland Career Framework Guidance [31], the Chief Nursing Officer Directorate and Health Workforce were eager to support the consistent and sustainable implementation of ANP in Scotland. This approach was linked to the development of the Advanced Practice Toolkit [30]. The Advanced Nursing Practice Tool Kit (http://www.advancedpractice.scot.nhs.uk) supports decision-making and planning based on the needs of patients and service. Furthermore, it draws together a body of work around an advanced level of nursing practice that states this level of practice reflects a particular benchmark above "Senior" level and below "Consultant" level on the Scottish career development ladder. The Toolkit sets out a consensus position on level of practice and offers an extensive array of tools and resources to support development and implementation of ANP. In connection to The Toolkit, the Scotland Career Framework Guidance [31] recommends that when considering if the option of an APN role is the best fit to meet the needs of patients that nursing directors, healthcare planners, and key stakeholders take into consideration service needs, education needs of the entire healthcare workforce, anticipated impact of introducing APN roles along with views of sustainability, and a robust governance/accountability scheme [31].

The Chief Nursing Officer (CNO) for Scotland, the CNO's for the other three countries of the United Kingdom (England, Northern Ireland, and Wales) and the UK Modernising Nursing Careers Coalition have all endorsed the Advanced Practice Toolkit and support clear guidance on advanced level nursing practice to be disseminated. As a result, NHS Wales (2009) accepted the principles contained within the Scottish Government Health Department's Advanced Practice Toolkit [30] to develop a framework structured to reflect key issues from the Scottish Toolkit [23].

6.1.3.4 Ireland: A Dual Credentialing Framework

In 1998, the Report from the Commission on Nursing: A Blueprint for the Future [32] recommended the establishment of the National Council for Nursing and Midwifery (NCNM) with one of its functions being the development of advanced nursing and midwifery posts and persons in Ireland. The Commission on nursing recognized that promotional opportunities for nurses and midwives wanting to remain in clinical practice should be open and recommended a three-step clinical career path in nursing and midwifery, one of which was advanced practice. In addition, in order to use the title advanced nurse practitioner (ANP) or advanced midwife practitioner (AMP), the nurse or midwife must be appointed and approved for a specific clinical post [8]. The ANP or AMP appointment follows a needs assessment, preparation of the clinical site, and accreditation of the site by the Nursing and Midwifery Board of Ireland (NMBI).

Ireland is one of the few countries currently requiring clearly defined documentation for both the development of the ANP/AMP along with the position and site where the ANP/AMP will be employed [20]. Both (post and ANP/AMP) are subject to regulatory body accreditation or oversight. The Nursing and Midwifery Board of Ireland (http://www.NMBI.ie) is the independent statutory body that regulates the nursing and midwifery professions in Ireland with its functions defined in the "Nurses and Midwives Act: 2011" [9, 10]. Over a 10-year period, 2001–2010, the NCNM (Nursing Council of Nursing and Midwifery) approved 154 Advanced Practice Posts and accredited 95 Advanced Nurse/Midwife Practitioners (ANP/AMP). In 2010, the Department of Health transferred the area of advanced practice from NCNM to An Bord Altranais, now referred to as NMBI (Nursing and Midwifery Board of Ireland). With the transfer from NCNM to NMBI, this agency now receives, reviews, and approves applications for the potential site for service delivery and for the ANP/AMP.

Documents provided to NMBI contain advanced practice role specification, job description, and site preparation details of the advanced practice posts. Site preparation includes criteria for the job title, title use, registration details, reporting relationships, location, background, and purpose of the post. In addition, documents must include a description of responsibilities for the ANP/AMP that cover clinical practice, level of autonomy, and practice expertise. The Director of Nursing of the clinical site seeking approval for the post presents information on post requirements, case load, and referral pathways to and from the ANP/AMP, scope of practice, working relationships, decision making autonomy, and competence maintenance. The Notary/Public Commission for Oaths notarizes documentation [4].

Standards and Requirements for Advanced Practice (Nursing) and Standards and Requirements Advanced Practice (Midwifery), based on the interim report WGAP 2014 [32], are due for publication later in 2016. In advance of this, NMBI has made a number of changes:

- Established a new interim revalidation process.
- All advanced practice forms have been reviewed and updated.
- Guidelines for advanced practice portfolios have been updated.
- Updated the guidelines in relation to advanced practice posts.

Expectations are that criteria for registration will change, specifically postregistration experience is being reduced. The issue of re-accreditation and portfolio development has been under review. The core concepts for advanced practice are also being extended. In the past the advanced practitioner could only work in a specific healthcare facility accredited by NMBI. This is likely to change, and a Registered Advanced Nurse practitioner will be eligible to apply to any healthcare facility they wish, i.e., approval of the post is now being separated from the person who is the ANP/AMP (K. Brennan, 21 May 2016, personal communication).

Begley et al. [3], in conducting a systematic evaluation of ANP/AMP in Ireland that also included a comprehensive literature review, emphasized that the complexity of identifying the distinctive nature of advanced practice should not be underestimated. Ireland, with nearly 20 years experience developing advanced nursing and midwifery roles, has taken the lead with a unique framework of dual credentialing and has also demonstrated the changes that take place following reassessment and evaluation of the initial regulatory process.

6.2   Credentialing

Credentialing processes and procedures refer to the mechanisms that officially regulate ANP and the individual APN. They include but are not limited to the assignment of degrees, authorization, endorsement, certification, licensure, accreditation, and registration. The methods chosen are usually connected to a country's regulatory traditions and agency resources in addition to what level is determined to be necessary to authorize the nurse to work within a scope of practice for an APN but beyond the scope of practice for a generalist nurse. Agencies and government departments will likely develop criteria and procedures to meet the expectations and prerequisites of legislation, public health/ministry of health departments, and the public (Gardner et al. [7]). All of these factors contribute to the way ANP is defined, credentialed, and put into practice.

The final choices for regulating or credentialing APNs depend on the regulatory environment of the region, country, or setting developing the credentialing processes. The following issues should be considered:

- Perceived potential and level of risk or harm to the consumer
- Potential benefit to the consumer
- Depth of specialized and advanced knowledge required
- Skills and abilities needed for practice
- Degree of autonomy expected of the role
- Extensiveness of the defined scope of practice

(Based on NCSBN [21])

Section 6.2.1 defines credentialing terminology and describes methods to consider when establishing a credentialing process for the APN.

6.2.1 Accreditation, Certification, Licensure, Registration, Endorsement

Various approaches are considered relevant for APN regulation and credentialing processes. In addition, credentialing may involve several steps (e.g., certification + licensure + registration) before a nurse can be declared to have full authority to practice as an APN. Some of the commonly used mechanisms are described below [12, 14]:

- *Licensure*: The use of licensure originates from the practice of creating standards for protection of the public [12]. Based on criteria of attaining a designated level of education and competency to practice within a defined scope, licensure is the most restrictive type of credentialing. Licensure grants the authority to practice. The validation processes to obtain the license ensures that the APN has met predetermined standards and is qualified to practice within a specified scope. It is generally used within a regulatory system that prohibits practice without a license.
- *Certification*: A time-limited formal process (examination, portfolio, or panel review of the applicant by clinical experts) used to validate an individual's knowledge, skills, and abilities. It can be voluntary or used as a requirement in the process to obtain an APN license. A nongovernmental agency or professional body usually conducts the process.
- *Registration*: Registration is a system whereby an individual's name is entered into an official register for persons who have specific qualifications. A register is maintained and monitored by a regulatory agency or official governmental department. If a country stipulates title protection for the APN, the person assigned the country designated title is registered as a method of identifying the APN. Registration is not a validation of competence and is usually the aspect of credentialing that requires renewal periodically for the APN to continue to practice.
- *Accreditation*: A process of review and approval by a qualified agency whereby a program, institution, or particular service is granted time-limited recognition having met predetermined criteria and standards.

- *Endorsement*: The use of endorsement as a requirement for entry into advanced practice stipulates criteria that must be met to be eligible for endorsement [1]. Criteria can include an unrestricted general nurse license, clinical leadership in a specified area, demonstrated competence, and completion of required qualifications as determined by an official regulatory agency within the country. Completion of the endorsement process authorizes the APN to function in an advanced clinical role (Australian Health Practitioner Regulation Agency/Nursing Midwifery Board Australia https://www.ahpra.gov.au/).

Regulatory terminology can mean different things in different countries leading to misunderstanding and misconception of the intent of the expressions. When assessing any one country's credentialing system, it is necessary to confirm what is involved in becoming credentialed, including the rights and protections that it includes. One issue that arises in reviewing credentialing processes is whether professional associations, governmental agencies, or other regulatory entities should establish the professional regulatory mechanisms. In Thailand the Nursing Council is the certifying agent and the credentialing authority [29]. A joint approach has been adopted by South Korea. The Ministry of Health and Welfare is the credentialing authority and has appointed the Korea Accreditation Board of Education to conduct the certification examinations for the APN [17, 18].

Credentialing can be considered mandatory or voluntary based on the established standards and requirements for the APN in the country and/or region. An education program for APNs may design a competency based and outcome focused curriculum that includes methods that ensure that the APN graduate has passed an assessment of professional knowledge including concrete clinical skills and complex decision making relevant to their practice focus. Initial appraisal of competency can be assessed through methods such as written examinations, OSCE (objective structured clinical examination), portfolio, and self-assessment.

Continued competency can be assessed through recertification and other compulsory processes. Under these circumstances the requirements are considered mandatory. When competence maintenance is viewed as voluntary, credentialing is viewed as simply a professional responsibility. Section 6.3 discusses issues to bear in mind when defining competence maintenance for APNs.

6.3   Maintaining Competence

Maintenance of professional competency or competence maintenance is a lifelong process of documenting professional accomplishments and activities. Mandatory competency maintenance is often a requirement for relicensure and ongoing credentialing for healthcare professionals including APNs. However, it is not clear that systems or methods intended to validate continued professional competence are successful in their intent to equip healthcare professional to maintain competence and keep up with advances in practice [16].

A number of factors have been identified as contributing to an inadequate demonstration that competence maintenance ensures quality professional practices [16]. The limitations include:

- Excessive reliance on lecture format and designated hours of learning rather than acquired knowledge or competence
- Limited attention placed on individuals meeting learning needs through self-assessment and self-directed learning
- Promotion of interprofessional collaboration or efforts to improve systems is weak
- Inadequate assistance for practitioners who want to assess and improve practice

Traditionally, under the continuing education model, value is measured by time spent attending a course such as a standard classroom lecture, workshop, or online offering. Competence maintenance in a continuing competence model calls for valuing activities based on a variety of factors beyond time. This perspective can include traditional options but broadens the choices that could be considered for maintaining competence. The range of choices could include: participation in or conduct of research, writing for publication, mentoring of APN students, clinical instructor, in-service teaching, structured interactive activities (e.g., group study), simulation, and participation in leadership functions (e.g., Board and Committee work). A move to interdisciplinary offerings at conferences, courses, workshops, and online learning has increased the variety of choices available. Competence maintenance also includes verification that the APN is clinically current and competent through regular practice in an identified clinical setting that includes identified hours in that clinical practice [12].

Criteria for maintaining competence are commonly linked to the APN scope of practice and/or focus area, identified competencies, and certification/licensure requirements. The timing cycle (commonly 5–8 years), documentation of accomplishments, and audit is typically determined by the credentialing bodies/authorities. If a written examination, generally called a certification exam, is utilized for the initial competency assessment, there is usually an option to retake the written examination to maintain certification. Standardization of competency assessment and reassessment processes is believed to be fundamental to ensuring the credibility of ANP [22].

In 2004, the Nursing Council of New Zealand established a Continuing Competence Framework (CCF) [26] with the intent to provide a mechanism to ensure nurses are competent to practice their profession. The Council has the authority to decline to issue an annual practice certificate (APC) if the applicant has failed to meet the required standard. The standards of competence expect a healthcare practitioner to practice within their scope of practice. In New Zealand, the four legislated scopes of practice for nurses (including nurse practitioner) each have their own set of competencies and standards and are expected to:

- Provide evidence of ongoing professional practice
- Provide evidence of ongoing professional development
- Provide evidence of meeting the Council's stipulated competencies for nursing scope of practice [27]

After reviewing the issue of continuing competence, the Nursing Council of New Zealand (2010) concluded that standards for entry level nursing competencies are clear while those for continued competence are not. Based on this report, one recommendation is for the NCNZ to provide a clear and more comprehensive definition of competence maintenance and the status of self-declaration assessment and the evidence needed to validate accomplishments.

Conclusion

This chapter describes the significance of professional regulation and credentialing in establishing as well as supporting the legitimacy of advanced practice nurses within healthcare systems and the healthcare workforce. Examples of professional regulatory frameworks and models are provided to offer guiding principles to inform and facilitate development of standards relevant to advanced nursing practice. Healthcare reform and changes within nursing communities and the nursing culture are leading the way for an era of progressive change that promotes a maturing of the discipline. Notable progress continues to be made internationally in the development of professional regulation supportive of the emerging diversity in advanced nursing practice. In addition, countries with longer histories of experience with advanced nursing roles demonstrate that sustainability of advanced nursing practice is linked to professional regulation and standard setting. All of these events suggest a bright future for the discipline and for nurses working at an advanced level in providing healthcare services.

References

1. Australian Government Department of Health (2012) Accessed 13 Apr 2016 from http://www.health.gov.au/internet/main/publishing.nsf/Content/work-nurse-prac
2. Barton TD, Bevan L, Mooney G (2012) Advanced nursing 2: a governance framework for advanced nursing. Nurs Times 108(25):22–24
3. Begley C, Murphy K, Higgins A, Elliott N, Lalor J, Sheerin F, Coyne I, Comiskey C, Normand C, Casey C, Dowling M, Devane D, Cooney A, Farrelly F, Brennan M, Meskell P, MacNeela P (2010) An Evaluation of Clinical Nurse and Midwife Specialist and Advanced Nurse and Midwife Practitioner Roles in Ireland (SCAPE). National Council for the Professional Development of Nursing and Midwifery in Ireland, Dublin
4. Carney M (2014, updated 2016) Advanced practice literature review report to NMBI (Nursing Midwifery Board Ireland). Author: Nursing and Midwifery Board (NMBI) Dublin
5. Council for Healthcare Regulatory Excellence (2008) Advanced practice: Report to the four UK health departments. Unique ID 17/2008
6. Department of Health (DH) (2006) Modernising nursing careers: setting the direction. Edinburgh: Scottish Executive. Accessed 19 Apr 2016 from http://www.gov.scot/resource/doc/146433/0038313.pdf
7. Gardner G, Carryer J, Dunn S, Gardner A (2004) Report to Australian Nursing & Midwifery Council: Nurse Practitioner Standards Project, Australian Nursing Council, Canberra
8. Government of Ireland (1998) Report of the commission on nursing: a blueprint for the future. The Stationery Office, Dublin
9. Government of Ireland (2011) Nurses and Midwives Act: 2011. The Stationery Office, Dublin
10. Government of Ireland (2011) Strategic framework for role expansion of nurses and midwives: promoting quality patient care. The Stationery Office, Dublin

11. Hamric AB (2014) A definition of advanced practice nursing. In: Hamric AB, Hanson CM, Tracy MF, O'Grady ET (eds) Advanced practice nursing: an integrative approach, 5th edn. Elsevier Saunders, St. Louis, pp. 67–85

12. Hanson CM (2014) Understanding regulatory, legal, and credentialing requirements. In: Hamric AB, Hanson CM, Tracy MF, O'Grady ET (eds) Advanced practice nursing: an integrative approach, 5th edn. Elsevier Saunders, St. Louis, pp 557–578

13. International Council of Nurses (ICN) (2001) ICN credentialing framework. Unpublished manuscript. Geneva: Author

14. International Council of Nurses (ICN) (2005) ICN regulatory terminology. Geneva: Author. Accessed 25 Apr 2016 from http://www.icn.ch/images/stories/documents/networks/ Regulation/Regulation_Terminology.pdf

15. International Council of Nurses (ICN) (2008) The scope of practice, standards and competencies of the advanced practice nurse, ICN Regulation Series. Author: ICN, Geneva.

16. Jhpiego (2014) Health Care Professional and Occupational Regulation Toolkit. Accessed 10 May 2016 from http://reprolineplus.org/resources/health-care-professional-and-occupational-regulation-toolkit

17. Kim DD (2003) The APN in Korea. Oral presentation at ICN conference. Geneva

18. Korean Accreditation Board of Nursing Education (KABONE) (2016) Accessed 18 Apr 2016 from http://kabon.or.kr/eng/index.php

19. Ministry of Health – New Zealand (MOH-NZ) (2002) Nurse practitioners in New Zealand. Author, Wellington

20. National Council for the Professional Development of Nursing and Midwifery (NCNM) (2008) Framework for the establishment of advanced nurse practitioner and advanced midwife practitioner posts. 4th edn. Accessed 26 May 2016 from https://www.pna.ie/images/ncnm/ ANPFramewrk%20(data%20prot%20version%20feb09).pdf

21. National Council of State Boards of Nursing (NCSBN) (2002) Regulation of advanced practice nursing: 2002 National Council of State Boards of Nursing position paper. Accessed 14 Apr 2016 from http://www.ncsbn.org

22. National Council of State Boards of Nursing (NCSBN) (2008) Consensus model for APRN Regulation: Licensure, accreditation, certification and education. Accessed 14 Apr 2016 from http://www.ncsbn.org/index.htm

23. National Leadership and Innovation Agency (2010) Framework for advanced nursing, midwifery and allied health professional practice in Wales. Accessed 19 Apr 2016 from http:// www.wales.nhs.uk/sitesplus/documents/829/NLIAH%20Advanced%20Practice%20 Framework.pdf

24. Nursing and Midwifery Council (NMC) (2008) The code: standards of conduct, performance and ethics for nurses and midwives. Author, London

25. Nursing and Midwifery Council (NMC) (2016) The code: standards of conduct, performance and ethics for nurses and Midwives. Retrieved 19 Apr 2016 from https://www.nmc.org.uk/ standards/code/

26. Nursing Council of New Zealand (NCNZ) (2004) Continuing competence framework. Nursing Council of New Zealand, Wellington

27. Nursing Council of New Zealand (NCNZ) (2010) Evaluation of the continuing competence framework. Nursing Council of New Zealand, Wellington: New Zealand

28. Nursing Council of New Zealand (NCNZ) (2015) Decision on nurse practitioner scope of practice and further consultation 2015. Retrieved 17 Apr 2016 from http://www.nursingcouncil.org. nz/Publications/Consultation-documents/Decision-on-nurse-practitioner-scope-of-practice-and-further-consultation-2015

29. Schober M, Affara F (2006) Advanced nursing practice. Blackwell Publishing Ltd., Oxford

30. Scottish Government (2008) Supporting the development of Advanced Nursing Practice – a toolkit approach. Accessed 19 Apr 2016 from http://www.advancedpractice.scot.nhs.uk/

31. Scottish Government (2010) Advanced nursing practice roles: guidance for NHS boards. Author, Edinburgh

32. WGAP (2014) Draft Interim Report WGAP (Working Group Advanced Practice). NMBI, Dublin. Accessed 24 May 2016 from http://www.nmbi.ie/ECommerceSite/media/NMBI/ WGAP-draft-interim-report.pdf

Challenges and Strategies

7

Abstract

The process of integrating advanced practice nursing roles into the healthcare workforce and diverse healthcare settings is a dynamic process characterized by constant change, alterations in service delivery, and progress toward a new era in nursing practice. The nature of these changes is met with both enthusiasm and skepticism. This chapter discusses reactions of other healthcare professionals and institutions to the introduction of advanced nursing practice. Views and dialogue on transformative and interprofessional education to facilitate collegial relations are discussed. Public perception and understanding of healthcare provided by advanced practice nurses is explored.

Keywords

Interprofessional • Intraprofessional • Transformative education • Public acceptance

The process of integrating advanced practice nursing (APN) roles into the healthcare workforce and diverse healthcare settings is a dynamic process characterized by constant change, alterations in service delivery, and progress toward a new era in nursing practice. The nature of these changes is met with both enthusiasm and skepticism. This chapter discusses reactions of other healthcare professionals to the introduction of advanced nursing practice (ANP) as a healthcare professional. Views and dialogue on transformative and interprofessional education to facilitate collegial relations are discussed. Public perception and understanding of healthcare provided by APNs is explored.

7.1 Professional Conflict

Points of view on the outcomes of APNs providing care similar to physicians seem to vary depending on whether the source of the surveys, studies, and publications originates from medical associations or nursing organizations. Even though APNs provide services that at times appear to overlap with what has been traditionally associated with physician services, the healthcare provided by APNs are distinctive to APN practice. Commonly, the differences of opinion as to the benefits of APN roles arise between representatives of medicine and nursing. Donelan et al. [20] suggest that the "turf war" should not be seen as unexpected. According to surveys conducted by medical associations [1, 2], there emerges a perspective that physicians provide better care when physicians and APNs provide the same service. This conclusion contrasts with other studies that demonstrate that care by APNs is similar to or better than physicians when providing the same service ([30, 37, 42, 44]). Results of a study by Donelan et al. [20] found that while the majority of physicians participating in their survey felt physicians provide better care, the majority of APN participants held the opinion that APNs would provide better care. In addition, to these incongruent perspectives, physicians and APNs had disparate views and professional perspectives of the APN role and scope of practice.

In spite of extensive literature ([30, 37, 42, 44, 45]) that supports the effectiveness of APNs to provide competent healthcare services, especially in primary healthcare, the opposing stance cites the longer and more rigorous training by physicians versus APNs and thus suggests that APNs are incapable of providing the same levels of quality and safe care as physicians [2]. On the other hand, there are physicians who recognize that the education is simply different and value the APN as a healthcare professional. A common theme reported by Donelan [20] that appears to fuel the physician/APN conflict is lack of knowledge by physicians and other healthcare professionals of the APN scope of practice, along with the depth and extent of knowledge acquired by this person. Additionally, it was also pointed out that the traditional hierarchal model of practice tends to promote medical dominance and thus limits effective teamwork and collaboration. A collaborative model is challenging if some physicians believe that APNs lack competence to provide the quality of care they would expect of a collaborator and colleague. At the policy level, in discussions regarding the APN scope of practice, some legislators and decision makers support the APN role and others back the position of medical organizations that oppose a broadened scope of practice for nurses [26].

These contrasting views imply that interdisciplinary conversations are needed to appreciate one another's roles and capabilities [22]. Findings from a focus group of general practitioners in England [52] identified threats to general practitioner status including job and financial security, nursing capabilities including training and scope of responsibility, and structural/organizational issues as barriers to accepting APNs. The study confirmed a need to develop a better understanding of the potential value of advanced nursing roles in general practice and how they will be positioned within the healthcare structure. This contrast in perspectives also highlights the need to provide evidence of APN sensitive outcomes.

7.1.1 Nursing

Students in APN programs and new graduates are not entirely surprised to experience some resistance from physicians when they proceed to implement the role. What is a surprise are intraprofessional boundary issues with other nurses [16]. The varying demands of the role and role overlap between nursing and medicine were found to contribute to experiences of intrapersonal dissonance [8], and it seems that problems among other categories of nursing remain even when relationships improve [23]. However, study findings regarding nurses' views of APN roles are mixed. In a study conducted in a hospital setting, nurses were worried that increased hierarchy within nursing will result from the introduction of APN roles [13]. This perception arises even when such a formal hierarchy among nurses does not exist [47]. Other studies found nurses had a positive attitude about what the APN could bring to a ward or unit, and over time the nurses saw the APNs as a resource and ceased to view them as a threat [27, 32, 34, 38].

Promoters of ANP in New Zealand anticipated dissent over interprofessional boundaries between APNs and physicians but were surprised by intraprofessional conflict between nurses [33]. A lack of understanding of the APN role by nursing colleagues was reported as a contributor to the friction [15, 29, 47]. Nursing leaders voiced concerns that APNs are seen as cheap physician substitutes thus losing the unique nature of the nursing profession [9, 16]. However, a survey conducted in the United Kingdom with 1,201 nurse practitioner respondents found that almost all (98 %) reported nursing skills as important to their practice and very few (8 %) considered their role to be that of a "mini-doctor" [3]. Additional studies [18, 19, 35] identify role ambiguity as a pivotal barrier to APN implementation with the most surprising resistance occurring with nursing colleagues. Roodbol [46] supported this contention and emphasized that on the one hand, the APN is expected to be a nurse; on the other hand, role expectations align the nurse with medicine. Role ambiguity appears to lead to role conflict when expectations are perceived to be contradictory [8]. Repeatedly, the importance of clearly defining and articulating each nursing role and scope of practice within a healthcare setting when integrating APN roles is emphasized [12, 25].

7.1.2 Medicine

Whether physicians are seen as champions for ANP or opponents, organized medical groups repeatedly fail to support ANP in the process of development and implementation of the roles. In a 32-country survey conducted by Pulcini et al. (2010), 83 % of the respondents named organized medical groups as opposing the APN role with 67 % of respondents noting that individual doctors opposed the role. In contrast, Heale and Rieck Buckley [28] reported that the majority of respondents in their study indicated that they did not experience opposition from other healthcare providers, but if opposition did occur, it was usually from physicians.

A view that APNs are in competition with physicians appears to arise from a stance that all healthcare is an extension of medicine therefore leading to misunderstanding when APNs see themselves as autonomous healthcare professionals [11]. Interprofessional conflict is rooted also in the perception that the APN poses an economic threat, a lack of experience of working together, and a history of traditional physician/nurse hierarchical structures [8]. Way et al. [50], in investigating shared responsibilities between physicians and APNs, found that APNs were underutilized with respect to curative and rehabilitative care with little evidence of collaborative management. In addition, findings from this study identified the inability of medicine to share responsibility, lack of interdisciplinary education, and lack of familiarity with the APN scope of practice. However, regardless of prevailing opinion, in most countries, physicians are viewed as the gatekeeper to the provision of healthcare services; thus, seeking support from medical professionals is central to a successful ANP initiative. The next two sections offer suggestions for resolving aspects of inter- and intraprofessional tension and strain. (See also Chapter 5, Role and Practice Development, for further discussion and strategies related to the issues of inter- and intraprofessional relations.)

7.1.2.1 Interprofessional Education and Experience

In attempting to reach a better understanding among professionals providing healthcare services, literature suggests that APNs and physicians should learn beneficial behavioral patterns to ease conflict and support collaboration ([36], Bailey et al. 2006). Nancarrow [43] in studying role boundaries in intermediate care teams with services provided by a variety of healthcare workers found that practitioners were not threatened by overlapping roles and concluded that role overlap can enhance healthcare professionals' confidence in their own area of expertise. Consistent with other studies on interprofessional collaboration, this study recommended joint visiting, and sharing work practice in situations of role overlap had the potential for optimizing staff resources. Barrett et al. [4] confirmed that interprofessional collaboration contributed to positive outcomes for patients, providers, and healthcare systems and could be beneficial in overcoming interprofessional conflict.

DiCenso et al. [17] in commenting on APN educational standards suggest that all health professionals should address interprofessionalism. The suggestion is that interprofessional education could facilitate effective teamwork among healthcare professionals [39]. The constant narrative of medical privilege and the position of physicians as the centerpiece for all healthcare development appear to be only one prevalent theme. In order to provide a comprehensive perspective on contributing factors to fragmented healthcare, 20 professional leaders from medicine, nursing, and public health from diverse countries formed a Lancet Commission to look at the tendency of various professions to act in isolation from or even in competition with each other. One major conclusion from the findings of this commission was a recommendation to move from seeking professional credentials to achieving core competencies for effective teamwork in health systems [24]. Based on findings from the Lancet Commission, Meleis [40] makes the following recommendations to promote transformative and interprofessional education:

- Students, faculty/educators, and consumers of care work together in changing education programs.
- Develop curricula based on competencies that are driven by population needs.
- Use of innovative instructional approaches.
- Develop congruent strategies to evaluate students in interprofessional programs.
- Develop mechanisms for accreditation that reflect interprofessionalism.
- Educate for critical thinking, teamwork, and team leadership while utilizing and translating best practices.

Interprofessional education is more likely to be successfully implemented when each profession participates in development of these strategies and when APNs are grounded in their own professional field. The most essential is the need to invest in the time and resources needed to ensure a paradigm shift from healthcare services focused on care provided only by physicians and medical consultants to the inclusion of and collaboration with all healthcare professionals, including APNs. Meleis [41] emphasizes that goals of interprofessional education and collaborative practice may not be achieved until the isolated nature of professional identities and power differentials are addressed. Clearly, this will not happen overnight and requires forethought, patience, and perseverance along with a proactive a step-by-step approach [49].

7.2   Identifying APN Function in the Healthcare Workforce

A theme that dominates the international literature and impedes implementation of ANP is pervasive role ambiguity and lack of role clarity relevant to APN roles and their function within healthcare systems. Inclusive integration of APNs into healthcare systems implies that the APN roles are developed and utilized to their full potential. The provision of advanced accredited education, appropriate legislative and regulatory mechanisms, and planning need to come together to guide role development. Public awareness and leadership support are part of the optimal mix. However, the fundamental issue for most favorable integration is the need for role clarity and distinct definitions of how the APN will function in a healthcare setting in relation to other healthcare providers. In addition, it is vital that the APN is recognized by health workforce planners as a distinct category of healthcare worker in the nursing profession with a specified set of roles and competencies that can be used to put them in place as legitimate and necessary members of the healthcare team [17–19, 47].

There has been a scarcity of evidence to clearly identify ideal mechanisms for the best possible strategies for the implementation and evaluation of APN roles and related healthcare services. A systematic framework outlining steps for introducing and evaluating APN roles has been proposed by Bryant-Lukosius and DiCenso [5]. Since the launching of the PEPPA (participatory evidence-informed patient-centered process for APN role development) framework, this structured process has provided guidance for over 16 countries including the recent development of the PEPPA-Plus framework in Switzerland [7]. (An in-depth discussion of the PEPPA framework can be found in Chapter 5, Role and Practice Development.)

The emergence of ANP appears to be progressing to a new era where literature not only seeks to define, describe, and debate the dimensions of APN roles but also seeks to determine and promote optimal health outcomes for populations seeking care provided by APNs. The alignment of role clarity, definition of APN function, and identification of patient-centered care through evidence-informed decision making should appeal not only to healthcare professionals but to key stakeholders, government officials, regulators, nursing leaders, and policymakers. Persons in these key positions may not always comprehend the influence they exercise over various aspects of APN development and implementation. Advocates for ANP with a structured approach in hand have the possibility of offering strategic discussions on behalf of a rapidly expanding nursing discipline.

7.3   Public Acceptance

Findings from a systematic review of the literature 1990–2008 [44] revealed that not only was there a high level of evidence that APNs provide safe effective quality care to specific populations, but the findings also found a high level of evidence to support equivalent levels of patient satisfaction.

Additional literature supports these findings [30, 37, 42, 44, 45, 48]. In a survey conducted by the American Medical Association [2], results indicated that patients have a clear preference for care by a physician and are confused regarding the qualifications for providers who are not physician. However, given the source of this survey, it cannot be assumed that the results are impartial. Based on identified role ambiguity, patient participants suggested healthcare professionals should clearly identify their licensure, training, and expertise. Citing more extensive and in-depth education by family physicians compared to APNs, another medical survey concluded that patients prefer to see a physician [1]. In spite of the disparity in survey and study findings, no evidence was found to support statements that APNs provide inferior care or in any way endanger public or community health.

Even though there is evidence that demonstrates public acceptance and satisfaction with services provided by APNs is positive, not everyone has experienced care provided by an APN. In countries where physicians are viewed as the only acceptable healthcare provider, it requires a significant shift in attitude to consider service provision by an APN. The passage of time, exposure to the role, and clear information explaining the function of this nurse is critical. In a study investigating the benefits and challenges of introducing the role of advanced practice nurses in nurse-led out-of-hours care in Hong Kong, respondents viewed that benefits of the APN in Hong Kong outweighed the challenges. The greatest challenge was cited as lack of acceptance by other healthcare professionals. However, this challenge was compounded by the general publics' traditional attitudes to healthcare provision. The researchers indicated that education of the public regarding the APN role and services is crucial [10].

Professional boundary issues contribute to uncertainty for healthcare consumers when the meaning of APN scope of practice and expectations for care by APNs is unclear [14, 31]. Studies conducted in Australia [21] and Canada [6] identified the medical profession, fear of litigation, and government policies as barriers to implementation of the APN role. Bryant-Lukosius et al. [6] identified six themes that influence APN role implementation and that require consideration when seeking to interact with and educate the public:

- Confusion about APN terminology
- Failure to clearly define the roles
- Overemphasis on replacing or supporting physicians
- Underutilization of all spheres of APN practice
- Failure to address the contextual factors that can undermine the roles
- Limited utilization of an evidence-based approach to development, implementation, and evaluation

The themes identified by Bryant-Lukosius et al. [6] imply that the inability of the public to understand who the APN is combined with barriers to access APN services provides quite a hurdle to overcome. In addition, there is a scarcity of literature that explores in depth the consumer or public perspectives of care from APNs. Word of mouth, editorials, and narratives suggest that following positive experiences with care by APNs, the public becomes supportive and are strong advocates for ANP; however, research is needed to confirm this view.

7.3.1 How the Public Understands the Roles, Trends, and Multidisciplinary Collaboration Yet Overlapping Scopes of Practice

Literature demonstrates a growing presence of ANP worldwide. Repeatedly, the author has described a state of confusion that surrounds fundamental attempts to describe and understand the identity of APN roles. Rhetoric and dialogue on this topic inspires academics to publish professional literature, but it seems that conversation is practically ignored in the consumer press. When the terms "collaboration" and "choices" for healthcare services are mentioned, it is not clear what this means in the real world of healthcare as the public and community populations understand it. There is more to the cliché of a "turf war" between healthcare professionals than just a superficial disagreement. Collaboration among healthcare professionals or the lack thereof contributes to an image of fragmented care versus optimal healthcare service provision. In an era of healthcare reform and adjustments as to who should or will provide healthcare in diverse settings, the complexities of bringing clarity to the debate are immense. In addition, insurers or funders of healthcare services may be unwilling to reimburse care or management provided by an APN thus as a result denying the public access to this choice. However, regardless of the multilayered challenges, the author agrees with the opinion of Wilmont [51] in suggesting that the public, the consumers of healthcare services, deserve to have an understanding of the fundamental issues of these discussions.

Conclusion

This chapter discusses the complexities and multiple factors that present challenges between healthcare professionals when introducing APNs into the healthcare workforce. An optimal approach emphasizes clearly defining APN roles and their function within the healthcare workforce to ease inter- and intraprofessional collaboration and maximize the contributions of these nursing roles. Nursing and interprofessional education that includes innovative approaches to support collaborative practices is discussed. Finally, this chapter advocates for identifying teamwork based on population needs along with a comprehensive campaign to inform the public of issues that influence the best possible delivery of healthcare services that include not only APNs but a mix of healthcare professionals.

References

 1. American Academy of Family Physicians (AAFP) (2012) Patient perceptions regarding health care providers. Accessed 21 Apr 2016 from http://www.aafp.org/dam/AAFP/documents/about_us/initiatives/PatientPerceptions.pdf
 2. American Medical Association (AMA) (2010) AMA responds to IOM report on the future of nursing. Accessed 21 Apr 2016 from www.ama-assn.org/ama/pub/news/news/nursing-future-workforce.page
 3. Ball J (2007) Nurse practitioners 2006. The results of a survey of nurse practitioners conducted on behalf of the RCN nurse practitioner association. Royal College of Nursing (RCN), London
 4. Barrett J, Curran V, Glynn L, Goodwin M (2007) CHSRF synthesis: interprofessional collaboration and quality primary healthcare. Canadian Health Services Research Foundation, Ottawa
 5. Bryant-Lukosius D, DiCenso A (2004) A framework for the introduction and evaluation of advanced practice nursing roles. J Adv Nurs 48(5):530–540
 6. Bryant-Lukosius D, DiCenso A, Browne G, Pinelli J (2004) Advanced practice nursing roles: development, implementation and evaluation. J Adv Nurs 48(5):519–529
 7. Bryant-Lukosius D, Spichiger E, Martin M, Stoll H, Kellerhals SD, Fliedner M, Grossman F, Henry M, Herrmann L, Koller A, Schwendimann R, Ulrich A, Weibel L, Callens B, De Geest S (2016) Framework for evaluating the impact of advanced practice nursing roles. J Nurs Scholarsh 48(2):201–209. doi:10.1111/jnu.12199
 8. Brykczynski K (2014) Role development of the advanced practice nurse. In: Hamric AB, Hanson CM, Tracy MF, O'Grady ET (eds) Advanced practice nursing: an integrative approach, 5th edn. Elsevier, St. Louis, pp 95–116
 9. Carter AJE, Chochinov AH (2007) A systematic review of the impact of nurse practitioners on cost, quality of care, satisfaction and wait times in the emergency department. Canadian J Emerg Med 9(4):286–295
10. Christianson A, Vernon V, Jinks A (2013) Perceptions of the benefits and challenges of the role of advanced practice nurses in nurse-led out-of hours care in Hong Kong: a questionnaire study. J Clin Nurs 22(7-8):1173–1181
11. Cockerham AZ, Keeling AW (2014) A brief history of advanced practice nursing in the United States. In: Hamric AB, Hanson CM, Tracy MF, O'Grady ET (eds) Advanced practice nursing: an integrative approach, 5th edn. Elsevier Saunders, St. Louis, pp 1–26
12. Contandriopoulos D, Brousselle A, Carl-Ardy D, Perroux M, Beaulieu MD, Brault I, Kilpatrick K, D'Amour D, Sansgter-Gormley E (2015) A process-based framework to guide

nurse practitioners integration into primary healthcare teams: results from a logic analysis. BioMed Central. doi:10.1186/s12913-015-0731-5

13. D'Amour D, Morin C, Dubois C, Lavoie-Tremblay M, Dallaire C, Cyr G (2007) Évaluation de l'implantation du programme d'intéressement au titre d' infirmière praticienne spécialisée. Rapport de recherche présenté au Ministère de la Santé et des Services sociaux du Québec. Montréal Centre, Ferasi

14. Daly WM, Carnwell R (2003) Nursing roles and levels of practice: a frameworkfor differentiating between elementary, specialist and advanced nursing roles. J Clin Nurs 12(2):158–167

15. de Leon-Demare K, Chalmers K, Askin D (1999) Advanced practice nursing in Canada: has the time really come? Nurs Stand 14(7):49–54

16. DiCenso A, Bryant-Lukosius D (2010) Role of clinical nurse specialists and nurse practitioners in Canada: a decision support synthesis. Canadian Health Services Research Foundation, Ottawa

17. DiCenso A, Martin-Misener R, Bryant-Lukosius D, Bourgeault I, Kilpatrick K, DiCenso A, Bryant-Lukosius D, Martin-Misener R, Donald F, Abelson J, Bourgeault I, Kilpatrick K (2010) Factors enabling advanced practice nursing role integration role in Canada. Canadian J Nurs Leadership 23(Special Issue):211–238

18. Donald F, Kaasalainen S, Harbman P, Carter N, Kioke S, Abelson J, McKinlay RJ, Pasic D, Wasyluk B, Vohra J, Charbonneau-Smith R (2010) Advanced practice nursing in Canada: overview of a decision support synthesis. Canadian J Nurs Leadership 23(Special Issue):15–34

19. Donald F, Bryant-Lukosius D, Martin-Misener R, Kaasalainen S, Kilpatrick K, Carter N, Harbman P, Bourgeault I, DiCenso A (2010) Clinical nurse specialists and nurse practitioners: title confusion and lack of role clarity. Canadian J Nurs Leadership 23(Special Issue):189–210

20. Donelan K, DesRoches CM, Buerhaus P (2013) Perspectives on physicians and nurse practitioners on primary care practice. N Engl J Med 368:1898–1906. doi:10.1056/NEJMsa1212938

21. Elsom S, Happell B, Manias E (2008) Expanded practice roles for community mental health nurses in Australia: confidence, critical factors for preparedness and perceived barriers. Issues Ment Health Nurs 29(7):767–780

22. Fairman JA, Rowe JW, Hassmiller S, Shalala DE (2011) Broadening the scope of nursing practice. N Engl J Med 364(3):193–196. doi:10.1056/NEJMp1012121

23. Fawcett J, Newman DMI, McAllister M (2004) Advanced practice nursing and conceptual models of nursing. Nurs Sci Q 17(2):135–138

24. Frank J, Chan L, Bhutta ZA, Cohen J, Crisp N, Evans T, Fineberg HH, Garcia P, Pe Y, Kelley P, Kistnasamy B, Meleis A, Naylor D, Pablos- Mendez A, Reddy S, Scrimshaw S, Sepulveda J, Serwadda D, Zurayk H (2010) Health professionals for a new century: transforming education to strengthen health systems in an interdependent world. Lancet. 376(9756):1923–1958 doi:10.1016/S0140-6736(10) 61854-5

25. Griffiths H (2006) Advanced nursing practice: enter the nurse practitioner. Nurs BC 38(2):12–16

26. Hain D, Fleck LM (2014) Barriers to nurse practitioner practice that might impact healthcare redesign. Online J Issues Nursing. 19(2):Manuscript 2. doi:10.3912/OJIN.Vol19No02Man02

27. Harwood I, Wilson B, Heidenheim AP, Lindsay RM (2004) The advanced practice nurse-nephrologist care model: effect on patient outcomes and hemodialysis unit team satisfaction. Hemodial Int 8(3):273–282

28. Heale R, Rieck Buckley C (2015) An international perspective of advanced practice nursing regulation. INR 62(3):421–429. doi:10.1111/inr.12193

29. Higuchi KA, Hagen B, Brown S, Zeiber MP (2006) A new role for advanced practice nurses in Canada: bridging the gap in health services for rural older adults. J Gerontol Nurs 32(7):49–55

30. Horrocks S, Anderson E, Salisbury C (2002) Systematic review of whether nurse practitioners working in primary care can provide equivalent care to doctors. Br Med J 324(734):819–823

31. International Council of Nurses (ICN) (2008) The scope of practice, standards and competencies of the advanced practice nurse. ICN Regulation Series. ICN, Geneva

32. Irvine D, Sidani S, Porter H, O'Brien-Pallas L, Simpson B, McGillis Hall I, Fraydon J, DiCenso A, Redelmeir D, Nagel I (2000) Organizational factors influencing nurse practitioners' role implementation in acute care settings. Can J Nurs Leadersh 13(3):28–35

33. Jacobs SH, Boddy JM (2008) The genesis of advanced nursing practice in New Zealand: policy, politics and education. Nurs Praxis in New Zealand, J Prof Nurs 24(1):11–22
34. Jensen I, Scherr K (2004) Impact of the nurse practitioner role in cardiothoracic surgery. Dynamics 15(3):14–19
35. Jones ML (2005) Role development and effective practice in specialist and advanced practice roles in acute hospital settings: systematic review and meta-synthesis. J Adv Nurs 49(2):191–202
36. Jones L, Way D (2004) Delivering primary health care to Canadians: Nurse practitioners and physicians in collaboration. Practice Component: Literature Review Report. Canadian Nurses Association and Canadian Nurse Practitioner Initiative, Ottawa
37. Lenz ER, Mundinger MO, Kane RL, Hopkins SC, Lin SX (2004) Primary care outcome in patients treated by nurse practitioners or physicians: Two-year follow-up. Medical Care Research and Review, 61(3):332–351. doi: 10.1177/1077558704266821
38. Macdonald M, Schreiber R, Davidson H, Pauly B, Moss L, Pinelli J, Regan S, Crickmore J, Hammond C (2005) Moving through harmony: exemplars of advanced nursing practice for British Colombia. Can J Nurs Leadersh 20:39–44
39. Martin-Misener R, Bryant-Lukosius D, Harbman P, Donald F, Kaasalainen S, Carter N, Kilpatrick K, DiCenso A (2010) Education of advanced practice nurses in Canada. Can J Nurs Leadersh. (Special Issue). pp 61–87
40. Meleis A (2011) Education of health professionals for the 21st century and its significance for nursing. Nursing & Midwifery links. The Global Network of WHO Collaborating Centres for Nursing and Midwifery Development. University of Sao Paulo. Ribeirao Preto College of Nursing, Sao Paulo
41. Meleis A (2016) Interprofessional education: a summary of reports and barriers to recommendations. J Nurs Scholarsh 48(1):106–112
42. Mundinger MO, Kane RL, Lenz ER, Totten AM, Tsai WY, Cleary PD, Shelanski ML (2000) Primary care outcomes in patients treated by nurse practitioners or physicians: a randomized trial. JAMA 283(1):59–68. doi:10.1001/jama.283.1.59
43. Nancarrow S (2004) Dynamic role boundaries in intermediate care services. J Interprof Care 18(2):141–151
44. Newhouse RP, Stanik-Hutt J, White KM, Johantgen M, Bass EB, Zangaro G, Wilson RF, Fountain L, Steinwachs PM, Heindel L, Weiner JP (2011) Advanced practice nurse outcomes 1990–2008: a systematic review. Nurs Econ 29(5):1–21
45. Pinkerton JA, Bush HA (2000) Nurse practitioners and physicians: patients' perceived health and satisfaction with care. J Am Acad Nurse Pract 12(6):211–217. doi: 10.1111/j.1745-7599.2000.tb00184.x
46. Roodbol P (2005) Willing o'-the-wisps, stumbling runs, toll roads and song lines: study into the structured rearrangement of tasks between nurses and physicians. Summary of doctoral dissertation. Unpublished
47. Schober M (2013) Factors influencing the development of advanced practice nursing in Singapore. Doctoral thesis, Sheffield Hallam University, Sheffield Hallam University archives. Accessed 30 Apr 2016 from http://shura.shu.ac.uk/7799/
48. Swan M, Ferguson S, Chang A, Larson E, Smaldone A (2015) Quality of primary care by APNs: a systematic review of equal or better outcomes for physiologic measures, patient satisfaction and cost. Int J Qual Healthcare 27(5):396–404
49. Tomasik J, Fleming C (2014) Lessons from the field: promising interprofessional collaboration practices. Robert Wood Johnson Foundation, Princeton
50. Way D, Jones L, Baskerville B, Busing N (2001) Primary health care services provided by nurse practitioners and family physicians in shared practice. Can Med Assoc J 165(9):1210–1214
51. Wilmont SS (2013) Doctors and nurse practitioners: beyond the turf wars. Colombia Journalism Review. The Second Opinion
52. Wilson A, Pearson D, Hassey A (2002) Barriers to developing the nurse practitioner role in primary care. Fam Pract 19(6):641–646

Career Paths, Clinical Career Ladders, and Professional Progression

8

Abstract

The development of advanced nursing practice and diverse advanced practice nursing roles along with the increased presence of this discipline signals a new era for nursing. This upsurge in visibility appears to be a way to enhance career prospects in the nursing profession. Successful integration of advanced practice nursing roles into the healthcare workforce includes promoting professional advancement. Creating a career path acknowledges advanced practice nursing contributions to healthcare settings, provides concrete recognition of this nursing role, and potentially leads to personal job satisfaction. This chapter explores multiple factors to bear in mind when considering developing a career pathway or clinical ladder that includes advanced practice nursing roles and advanced levels of practice. In addition, principles that form the foundation for professional progression are offered. Illustrations of country specific career pathways are described.

Keywords

Clinical ladder • Career pathway • Professional progression • Recognition

The development of advanced nursing practice and diverse advanced practice nursing roles along with the increased presence of this discipline worldwide signals a new era for nursing. This upsurge in visibility appears to be a way to enhance career prospects in the nursing profession [10]. Successful integration of APN roles into the healthcare workforce includes promoting professional advancement. Creating a career path acknowledges APN contributions to healthcare settings, provides concrete recognition of this nursing role, and potentially leads to personal job satisfaction [6]. This chapter explores multiple factors to bear in mind when considering developing a career pathway or clinical ladder that includes APN roles and level of practice. In addition, principles that form the foundation for professional progression are offered. Illustrations of country specific career pathways are described.

8.1   Adaptation to the Role

After the APN student completes an education program, the first year is focused primarily on developing clinical competence and refining role components based on theories acquired in the course/program. As the APN graduate begins practice, the journey has begun on the path toward professional success. A clinical career ladder or pathway inclusive of ongoing evaluation strategies that link the development of APN services to the healthcare setting while meeting individual professional aspirations of the individual is critical [1].

Formal support for healthcare professionals, especially in institutional settings, is often specific to physician and generalist nurses rather than specific to the unique nature of the APN role. In some situations this leaves the APN, especially those in the private sector, to independently negotiate issues such as promotion and salary increases. The consequence of depending on independent negotiations can result in uneven development in the roles, professional progress, and incentives sometimes within the same institutions, across institutions and the country. A career ladder/ path provides a means to effectively measure accomplishments and contributions within an institution and healthcare setting. In addition, a model for professional advancement such as a career ladder allows for role definition with clearer expectations and guidelines for ongoing professional growth. The ICN [8] position suggests that appropriate career development needs to include:

- A correlated system of education and professional development
- Established career structures (e.g., career ladder with different pathways)

To realize its full potential, ICN [8] defines career mobility in nursing as the movement of nurses to more advanced levels, different areas of nursing practice, or to positions in which different functions exist (e.g., advanced practice). The ICN position statement further asserts that career development must be supported and sustained by means of a defined educational system, recognized career structures (including career ladders) flexible enough to provide career mobility. Attributes of a career progression structure should include reward mechanisms such as recognition, advancement, and/or compensation/salary. In countries where unions negotiate these elements for APNs, it is vital that APN representatives educate them about the roles.

Career structures for nurses have traditionally been associated with education or management paths. Career ladders, where they exist, tend to designate more advanced levels of promotion to these fields with little advancement opportunity or incentive for nurses to remain and develop in clinically focused employment. The development of a clinical path that recognizes and rewards clinical nursing alongside management and education as a career progression opportunity is emerging as a strategy to promote and reward clinical excellence in order to encourage nurses to remain in a clinical role.

8.1.1 Creating Career Ladders/Professional Development Structures

One way of guiding nurses through career development is with a pathway or ladder to success and professionalism in nursing. The following four major steps present a basic foundation in developing a career path/ladder.

- Identifying the principles that underpin the decision-making concerning the structure of the career path/ladder
- Developing a consensus on defining the levels for career structure
- Establishing and defining the elements to be incorporated into the career structure, and developing
  - Template job descriptions based on defined scopes of practice and competency frameworks
  - Appropriate performance assessment tools
- Implementing the career structure within the system – achieving consensus, piloting, refining the clinical path prior to a systematic implementation nationwide with a continuous monitoring and evaluation plan

In constructing a career structure for professional progression a number of underlying principles can be used to guide development.

- Establish a standard that sets up one national career ladder/pathway.
- A clinical path is one of the possible paths to follow, e.g., clinical, education, administration, and research.
- Along with vertical progression consider horizontal mobility across different paths as a possibility, e.g., mobility move from a clinical to an educator path or vice versa, provided the criteria for the requirements are met.
- Comparable criteria used to define each path and across levels.
- Competence-based role requirements are based on scope of practice.
- Career advancement and promotion is based on demonstrated merit and health service needs.
- Performance appraisals are consistent with expected roles and responsibilities as defined in the job descriptions/scope of practice.

Defining the prerequisites of a career ladder is essential based on what is realistic in the country's current system. For example, requiring evidence of a certain level of education and or professional development that is unachievable will present an obstacle in implementation and reduce the credibility of the career structure. In the beginning, it may be optimal to define the criteria in broad terms and introduce flexibility into system requirements. As the professional development system matures and becomes more rigorous, these aspects can be refined according to the prevailing healthcare or nursing culture and environment.

8.1.2   Diversity in Advanced Nursing Practice Clinical Career Structures

Approaches to defining a clinical career structure relevant to ANP evolve based on country, institution [public versus private sector], and professional perspectives of what professional progression means. Two arrangements can be identified relevant to career progression for nurses [2]. One is linked to the benefits an individual gains in a defined APN role versus another view where advancement is defined in relation to how the role is placed within designated nursing levels in the healthcare system. In Ireland, the Report of the Commission on Nursing [7] was the catalyst for the introduction of a clinical career pathway that encompasses progression from staff nurse or staff midwife to clinical nurse specialist or midwife specialist to advanced nurse practitioner or midwife practitioner. A similar view of career progression is evident in Japan, Taiwan, and Thailand [3].

The Commission on Nursing in Ireland recognized that promotional opportunities should be available to nurses and midwives who want to remain in clinical practice and for that reason recommended a clinical career pathway leading from registration to clinical specialization to advanced practice. When established, the National Council for the Professional Development of Nursing and Midwifery developed a definition, core concepts, and competencies and requirements for the advanced nurse practitioner and advanced midwife practitioner [12]. One original aim in development of this framework was to retain expert nurses in direct patient care. This objective occurred against a background of healthcare service reform in the country. The development of this career pathway was part of the strategic development of overall health service needs and provides for standardized development of strategies for continued support of the role relative to health service needs versus the individual need of the advanced nurse practitioner. As an example of the aim to enhance nursing and midwife roles, this model is unique in that it is based on identified healthcare service needs in order for a site to prepare for the introduction of an APN. Once a clinical site has received approval and funding, an APN applicant must be approved for the post, thus the clinical pathway rests on a system of dual approval (see Sect. 6.1.3.3 for further discussion of the credentialing framework in Ireland).

In Singapore, clinical career progression for the APN is achieved based on progression from staff nurse (diploma/degree) > nurse clinician > senior nurse clinician > advanced practice nurse > Assistant Director of Nursing (clinical) > Deputy Director (clinical) ultimately resulting in the opportunity to seek a position of Director of Nursing if the individual progresses along this pathway [11]. The nurse can move through the various levels of nursing with appraisal and performance measured against criteria for each level; however, greater importance is assigned to administrative/managerial components that the individual nurse has achieved with limited support for sustainability in a clinically focused role [13].

Under the auspices of the United Kingdom wide Modernising Nursing Careers (MNC) initiative [5], a Toolkit approach was developed through the Chief Nursing Officer Directorate of the Scottish Government [15]. The framework and toolkit builds on earlier Scottish work and articulates how a structured nursing career framework could be used to support national healthcare priorities. As a result of the work done in Scotland, similar pathways, reflecting country specific national priorities, took place in England, Northern Ireland, and Wales. A focus was on establishing clarity and consistency regarding the key stages of the career framework to provide clear pathways for staff development, staff deployment, and service delivery. The Modernising Nursing Careers initiative provided an opportunity to structure a genuine career framework for nursing supporting forward movement throughout their career.

The Scottish initiative places ANP and the APN roles within a career structure and identifies steps for progression from staff support roles to advanced roles to consultant level and more senior posts, all levels requiring the appropriate education and evaluation to ensure that the candidate meets need of healthcare service delivery. The Advanced Nursing Practice Toolkit [15] is a UK-wide resource and has been endorsed by Chief Nursing Officers for all four countries (Scotland, England, Northern Ireland, Wales). In the National Health Service (NHS) Career framework ANP is at the designated career level – Level 7. In addressing payment for services, the framework suggests linking to the NHS Pay System (http://www.paymodernisation.scot.nhs.uk/afc/index.htm) that is intended to ensure fair pay and a clear system for career progression. This system is an attempt to ensure staff are paid on the basis of the jobs they are doing along with the knowledge and skills they utilize within their position underpinned by a job evaluation scheme matching jobs to national profiles for healthcare needs.

8.2 Linking Job Descriptions, Scopes of Practice, and Competencies

Country context will dictate an orientation either to the terms job descriptions or scopes of practice in reference to career paths or professional development. Adding to already noted confusion, sometimes the terms job descriptions and scopes of practice are used interchangeably [4]. However, literature suggests that job descriptions are institution-led descriptions of facility-level roles based on rules and policies. Job descriptions tend to be prescriptive written employer statements outlining the duties, purpose, and responsibilities of a job or position [4, 14]. Scope of practice is considered to be broader, multifactoral, multifaceted, and linked to advanced critical thinking, decision-making, and knowledge. The use of scope of practice varies but often includes actions, processes, and responsibilities of a healthcare professional who agrees to function consistent with a professional license and standard. In this chapter in reference to ANP and relevant career ladders/paths, reference is made most often to scopes of practice. (Refer to Chap. 3: Nature of Practice for an in-depth discussion of Scope of Practice for the APN.)

The scope of practice identifies and communicates the health worker's range of activities – roles, functions, responsibilities, activities, accountability, decision-making capacity, and authority. The scope and competencies relate to not only professional progression but to professional standards and policies. In a model provided by the Jhpiego Toolkit on healthcare professional and occupational scopes of practice, professional standards, policies, and procedures (SSPP) are linked in a logical manner with one being the foundation stone for another. Professional standards grow out of the definition of a profession's scope of practice. Competencies and standards are derived from an analytical process resulting in scope of practice definitions. The use of scope of practice as a foundation to inform health service delivery operational processes and those related to healthcare personnel management as in the construction of career ladders is likely to promote greater coherence and relevance in linking the various steps of career progression. (See Sect. 6.1.2 for further discussion of the SSPP model).

8.3   Performance Review and Evaluation

There are claims that clinical pathways and career ladders promote recruitment and retention of nurses. When developed and implemented in relation to ANP, the structure implies that there is performance review and evaluation of the APN. This can be viewed as a two-pronged process that: (1) refers to continuous professional development systems that are implementable, relevant, and career structures associated with a payment or reimbursement system for service provision (2) Links performance assessment to scope of practice and codes of professional practice. As noted in the previous section, using the SSPS (scopes of practice, professional standards, policies, and procedures) model to develop criteria for performance review and evaluation can provide a foundation [9]. However, there is a scarcity of literature on implementation of career development structures for ANP.

Conclusion

Career ladders and pathways are viewed as structures that facilitate career progression and associated differentiation of pay/salary, promotion, and/or benefits by defining different levels of clinical practice. Career progression for nursing, including advanced nursing practice, is beginning to be integrated into national healthcare frameworks linked to healthcare needs and priorities. The evidence base for the use or benefit of clinical ladders is fragmented and mainly based on narrative accounts. This chapter describes fundamental principles supportive of clinical career ladders and pathways; however, research and objective analysis is needed to fully determine the benefits of these structures, their relevance to advanced nursing practice, and optimal practices for implementation.

References

1. Bryant-Lukosius D, DiCenso A (2004) A framework for the introduction and evaluation of advanced practice nursing roles. J Adv Nurs 48(5):530–540
2. Buchan J (1999) Evaluating the benefits of a clinical ladder for nursing staff: an international review. Int J Nurs Stud 36(2):137–144
3. Chiang-Hanisko L, Ross R, Boonyanurak P, Ozawa M, Chiang L (2008) Pathways to progress in nursing: understanding career patterns in Japan, Taiwan and Thailand. OJIN 13(3)

4. Corazzini KN, Anderson RA, Rapp CG, Mueller C, McConnell E, Lekan D (2010) Delegation in long-term care: scope of practice or job description. Online J Issues Nurs 15
5. Department of Health (2006) Modernising nursing careers: setting the direction. Accessed 09 May 2016 from http://www.scotland.gov.uk/Publications/2006/08/31120554/0
6. Faris JA, Douglas MK, Maples DC, Berg LR, Thrallkill A (2010) Job satisfaction of advanced practice nurses in the Veterans Health Administration. JAANP 22(1):35–44. doi:10.1111/j.1745-7599.2009.00468.x
7. Government of Ireland (1998) Report of the Commission on Nursing: A blueprint for the future. Government of Ireland Publications, Dublin.
8. International Council of Nurses (ICN) (2007) Career development in nursing, position statement. ICN, Geneva
9. Jhipiego (2014) Health care professional and occupational regulation toolkit. Author: Jhpiego, an affiliate of Johns Hopkins University
10. MacDonald-Rencz S, Bard R (2010) The role for advanced practice nursing in Canada. Can J Nurs Leadersh 23(Special Issue):8–11
11. Ministry of Health Singapore (2012) Career tracks for nursing. Accessed 08 May 2016 from https://www.moh.gov.sg/content/moh_web/healthprofessionalsportal/nurses/career_practice/nursing_careers.html
12. National Council for the Professional Development of Nursing and Midwifery (NCNM) (2008) Framework for the establishment of advanced nurse practitioner and advanced midwife practitioner posts, 4th edn. NCNM, Dublin
13. Schober M (2013) Factors Influencing the Development of Advanced Practice Nursing in Singapore. Doctoral thesis. Sheffield Hallam University, Sheffield Hallam University archives. Accessed 4 Mar 2016 from http://shura.shu.ac.uk/7799/
14. Schuiling KD, Slager J (2000) Scope of practice: freedom within limits. J Midwifery Womens Health 45(6):465–471
15. Scottish Government (2008) Supporting the development of advanced nursing practice: a toolkit approach. Author: CNO Directorate, Scottish Government

Research

9

Abstract

As the discipline of advanced nursing practice matures attention on advanced clinical expertise remains the focus while additional core competencies such as leadership and research have become included when characterizing advanced practice nursing roles. Understanding research, the utilization of data and participation in the research process, especially as it provides evidence for effective practice, has become an integral component of educational programs and expected educational outcomes for an advanced practice nurse graduate. This chapter introduces research as a role competency for advanced nursing practice and discusses the essential nature of evidence-based practice. Examples of models and frameworks that support and encourage participation in research are provided. The chapter concludes with the profile of a university-based research center that educates, supports, and mentors advanced practice nurse participation in research.

Keywords

Evidence • Evidence-based practice • Research • Research center • Mentor

As the discipline of advanced nursing practice (ANP) matures attention on advanced clinical expertise remains the focus while additional core competencies such as leadership and research have become included when characterizing advanced practice nursing (APN) roles. The inclusion of research as a role component may vary on country context and the comparative significance in the roles of clinical nurse specialists versus other categories APNs. Understanding research, the utilization of data and participation in the research process, especially as it provides evidence for effective practice, has become an integral component of educational programs and expected educational outcomes for an APN graduate. Although APNs may not always be the principal investigators in a research study, there is an increased expectation of their participation in the research process. This chapter introduces research as a role competency for ANP and discusses the essential nature of evidence-based practice. Examples of models and frameworks that support and encourage participation in research are provided. In addition, the chapter concludes with the profile of

© Springer International Publishing Switzerland 2016
M. Schober, *Introduction to Advanced Nursing Practice*,
DOI 10.1007/978-3-319-32204-9_9

a university-based research center that educates, supports, and mentors APN involvement in research.

Documentation of the influence of APNs on healthcare provision appears to be improving, however, too often either the impact of the APN role is not evaluated or provision of care is not credited to the APN. 'Verifying APN contributions requires an assessment of the structures, processes, and outcomes associated with APN performance and the care delivery systems in which they practice' (Kleinpell and Alexandrov [9], p. 607). It is not within the scope of this chapter to explore all avenues of research and the research process. The intent of the author is to familiarize the reader with the significance of research and evidence-based practice as it relates to ANP and the nurse practicing in APN roles.

9.1   Evidence-Based Practice

Evidence-based practice is viewed as the incorporation of research findings (evidence) into clinical decision-making and delivery of care. Evidence-based data are also useful for development of practice guidelines [9] and to confirm the presence of outcomes associated with ANP. In explaining research-sensitive care as a sub-topic for evidence-based practice, Tracy [12] describes the manner in which the APN can use research findings that are relevant to clinical care. This approach considers the following to be essential for the APN:

- Reading research reports and summaries on a routine basis
- Informally assessing the reliability of the methods and findings
- Integrating knowledge to maintain current practice

(DePalma [4]; Tracy [12])

Evidence-based practice is a systematic method of translating research findings into practice. The APN research competency is increasingly being emphasized as the discipline of ANP becomes more established. DePalma [4] proposes that the APN integrates research competencies at two levels. At the basic level, as a student, the APN learns to understand and apply research skills. At the expanded level, the APN builds on these skills through actual participation and collaboration in the research process. Acquiring skills in the research process includes writing for publication and applying research findings into practice. Attaining this knowledge results from active participation and mentored guidance. (See Sect. 9.2 for an in-depth description of an advanced practice research center and their model for research mentorship). Sections 9.1.1 and 9.1.2 provide a model and resources for the conduct of research.

9.1.1   Joanna Briggs Institute Model

The Joanna Briggs Institute (JBI) regards evidence-based healthcare as a cyclical process and offers a model (see Fig. 9.1) for those who seek to gain evidence to

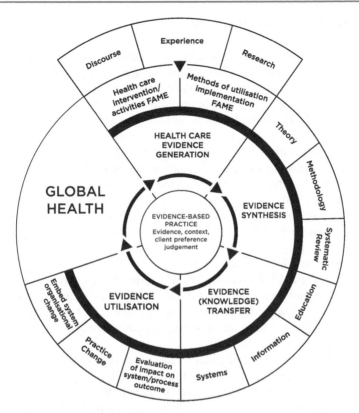

Fig. 9.1 Joanna Briggs Institute model for evidence-based practice (Access from http://www. joannabriggs.org/Jbl-approach.html)

demonstrate the diverse and numerous factors that impact on healthcare outcomes, health systems, and professional practice.

The Joanna Briggs Institute Model:

- Considers international evidence related to the feasibility, appropriateness, meaningfulness, and effectiveness of healthcare interventions (evidence generation)
- Includes these different forms of evidence in a formal assessment called a systematic review (evidence synthesis)
- Globally disseminates information in appropriate, relevant formats to inform health systems, health professionals, and consumers (evidence transfer)
- Has designed programs to enable the effective implementation of evidence and evaluation of its impact on healthcare practice (evidence utilization) (Accessed 02 May 2016 from http://joannabriggs.org/jbi-approach.html)

This model builds on the work of leaders in the field of evidence-based healthcare. The conceptual model attempts to emphasize the importance of healthcare evidence, its role, and its use within clinical practice settings worldwide [11].

9.1.2   Additional Research Resources

Evidence-based clinical decision-making is dependent on identifying research-based evidence. Expertise in searching the literature is essential to identify and retrieve appropriate studies. Electronic databases have revolutionized the ability to search for data albeit overwhelming at first as the APN gains experience and confidence to access the literature. It may be necessary to link to an institution, healthcare system, or library in some cases to access databases.

Administered by the USA National Library of Medicine, MEDLINE is the world's largest electronic database of health-related research and literature (http://medline.cos.com/). Articles originate from medicine, nursing, dentistry, and associated disciplines. The database is primarily organized around MESH words (medical subject headings); however, articles can also be retrieved using keywords that are in the title, abstract, or list of identifying keywords. The PubMed web page (http://www.ncbi.nlm.nih.gov/pubmed) provides free access to the MEDLINE database and will retrieve articles based on keywords.

The Cumulative Index for Nursing and Allied Health Literature (CINAHL) is the largest database for nursing and allied health literature including nursing journals that are not indexed in the MEDLINE database. Similar to MEDLINE, CINAHL database is available as a subscription service typically maintained by larger healthcare facilities and universities.

In addition to retrieving individual research reports, evidence-based data can be accessed through the Cochrane Library for Systematic Reviews. The Cochrane Library is part of the Cochrane Collaboration and is administered by a nonprofit organization, the Cochrane Working Group. The Cochrane Library contains multiple resources including the Cochrane Database of Systematic Reviews (http://www.cochrane.org/cochrane-reviews) and the Cochrane Register of Controlled Trials. Whenever available, the Database for Systematic Reviews includes a meta-analysis of data pooled from comparable studies. Reviews can be accessed by using keywords and obtained as a summary, standard report, or full report. The aim of the Cochrane Collaboration is to promote healthcare decision-making throughout the world that is informed by high-quality, timely research [10].

It may be obvious, but the author feels it needs to be stated that historical and existing practices based on tradition or clinical expertise alone may be harmful and even unethical if a practitioner continues to utilize unproven interventions, especially in the face of extensively researched topics available through today's healthcare resources. The examples provided in this chapter are not meant to identify an all-inclusive list of resources or databases but to introduce the significance of the emerging availability and reliance on databases and technology to obtain useful information. Due to the enormity of information and accessible data, strategies for searching electronic databases include accessing several databases along with consideration of assistance from a medical librarian or experienced researcher when available.

A case has been made for the importance of looking for and appraising the evidence; however, barriers to accessing and using the evidence need to be considered in order to develop strategies and competencies to enhance this skill. Houser and Oman [7] identify three categories of barriers:

- Overwhelming amount of evidence and contradictory findings at times
- Human factors
    - Lack of knowledge about and skills to use EBP
    - Negative attitudes regarding research and EBP
    - A view that research is only for medicine
- Lack of organization systems or infrastructure to support clinician use of evidence-based practice
    - Lack of authority of clinicians to make change in practices
    - Peer pressure to maintain same/or traditional practice
    - Lack of time
    - Lack of administrative support or incentives
    - Conflicting priorities
                        Conflicting priorities (Milner [10]; Houser and Oman [7])

Healthcare professionals and organizations are increasingly becoming evidence based and research focused. Agencies, governmental authorities, and professional organizations with the authority to promote and makes changes look to those in the field to provide data for ANP clinical practice, decision-making, requests for funding, and support for innovative ideas in provision of healthcare services. It is vital for APNs to address barriers that might be impeding a positive connection to a research informed, evidence-based professional presence. The model described in the following section provides an example of a resource center and concepts that facilitate APN interest and participation in research.

9.2   Conduct of and Participation in Research

The appeal for increased research associated with the international emergence of ANP and the identification of research as a role component implies that APNs have the flexibility to pursue this possibility. The reality of clinical workloads and additional responsibilities presents a context that makes this role component seem quite difficult. The following example provides a model of how this feature of ANP could be realized.

9.2.1   The Canadian Centre for Advanced Practice Nursing Research (CCAPNR) at McMaster University: A Resource and Model for Research Mentorship

To realize the full benefits of APN roles for patients, organizations, and health systems, healthcare leaders are recognizing the need to optimize the implementation of nonclinical role dimensions, such as research and evidence-based practice [3].

Although most APN educational programs include courses/modules related to research and/or evidence-based practice, this dimension of the role is widely known to be the most underdeveloped and underutilized [2, 5, 8].

Many advanced practice nurses report clinical responsibilities and service demands as taking precedence over nonclinical activities such as research. Even when employment agreements are in place that specify a percentage of work time for nonclinical activities, many advanced practice nurses are uncertain about how to start the process of leading research or evidence-based activities. Advanced practice nurses consistently report barriers to their involvement in research or evidence-based practice activities, including inadequate knowledge and skills, clinical role demands, lack of organizational support, and lack of appropriate mentors and resources [2].

To address these barriers, an innovative academic-practice partnership model was established in Canada to educate and mentor advanced practice nurses in leading and conducting point-of-care research, quality improvement, or evidence-based projects [6]. The aim of this initiative is to improve patient care by strengthening the capacity of advanced practice nurses to integrate research and evidence-based practice activities into their day-to-day practice. A description of the partnership's development, components, and evaluation follows.

9.2.1.1 Development and Components

Collaboration between an academic research team (Canadian Centre for Advanced Practice Nursing Research (CCAPNR) at McMaster University) and a large community hospital began when a team member conducted a research study within the hospital. This team member subsequently became a Nurse Scientist at this hospital with a directive to promote and develop APN research within the organization. An academic-practice partnership model was then created involving the Nurse Scientist, hospital administrators, advanced practice nurses, and CCAPNR to offer an applied research course delivered on-site by CCAPNR faculty. The initiative aimed to teach point-of-care providers how to lead research and evidence-based practice initiatives.

CCAPNR is a unique research enterprise in Canada, with a mandate to conduct research and build research capacity with respect to the effective use of APN roles through education, mentorship, and knowledge translation. CCAPNR faculty (nursing educators) members provided mentorship for participants to develop individual research or quality improvement (QI) projects during the course. Hospital administrators supported participants by covering the costs of the course and protected time off to attend the research course (two full day sessions, eight 3 h sessions).

Following this partnership, and building on what was learned during its development, a similar course arrangement was initiated with a healthcare organization in a different province. Eligible participants were again advanced practice nurses or nurses in leadership or professional practice roles who had: (1) completed a Master's degree with at least one research methods or statistics course, (2) identified a clinically relevant research question or QI or evidence-based practice issue, and (3) obtained agreement from their unit manager to provide time away from clinical work to participate in the course. Class size was limited to six to ten individuals to optimize peer interactions and collaborative learning and to ensure individualized education to build research competencies.

9.2.1.2 Course Format and Content
The course was adapted to a certificate course from a graduate level course designed specifically for advanced practice nurses and delivered nationally for 10 years. Depending on the organization, the course was delivered using on-site or distance learning modalities (email, web, and tele-conferencing). CCAPNR faculty (educators) led seminars specific to their areas of methodological research expertise. Teaching strategies included large group discussion, small group activities, peer review, and one-to-one consultation to develop participants' research competencies. The course format and assignments were designed to build competencies from qualitative, quantitative, evidence-based, and QI perspectives that could be applied to their proposal development process. This was reinforced by complementary serial assignments. All proposals were designed to be relevant to the participant's role and practice setting as well as organizational priorities for improving clinical care, professional practice, or service delivery. The goal was for each student to have a solid draft research proposal or project plan that would be further refined and submitted to an ethics board or funding agency following course completion.

CCAPNR faculty (nursing educators) developed the course manual utilizing baseline needs assessment results (i.e., participant survey and interviews) to identify participant priority goals and objectives. The Nurse Scientist participated in all sessions as the research champion and linkage between the organization, CCAPNR, and participants. The use of existing organizational resources that support research, QI, and evidence-based activities was encouraged through their integration in seminar activities (e.g., librarian services, decision-support staff, information management and QI services, research services). Class activities provided opportunities for peer support and feedback and problem solving to address individual barriers to research.

The course concluded with all participants delivering a scholarly presentation outlining their proposal to faculty (nursing educators), clinical program directors, and members of the hospitals' executive leadership team. The objective was to develop critical thinking about research and dissemination skills and to build confidence in seeking stakeholder feedback, buy-in, and project support.

9.2.1.3 Mentorship
Mentorship is essential for developing competencies and capacity to conduct research [1, 2]. Each participant was matched with a CCAPNR faculty (nursing educators) mentor to provide feedback on assignments and draft proposal, offer support and methodological guidance, identify relevant resources, and coach them through the process of leading research. Mentorship was important for helping participants develop skill sets and meet course timelines over a short 4-month time period. Mentors and participants interacted in a variety of ways (e.g., email, telephone, Skype, in person) at least twice each month during the course.

9.2.1.4 Evaluation

Irrespective of the type of hospital (e.g., community or university affiliated) where APNs worked, or how the course was offered (on-site versus distance format), the evaluation results were consistently positive. Students rated their overall satisfaction with the course as excellent (6.7 on a 1 (poor) to 7 (excellent) Likert scale) and there was a low attrition rate (10 %). Comparisons between pre- and postresponses in the combined dataset evaluating the extent to which participants performed specific activities and skills in their day-to-day practices yielded similar results. The largest improvements in post-course scores were for items related to confidence: in finding research evidence to support or improve current practice, to understand and evaluate the quality of research they read, to implement change based on research evidence in their practice, and to find the time to do research activities within their role [6].

Partnerships such as these, which are founded on a commitment to overcome research barriers in 'real world' practice settings, are encouraging. With all partners engaged, this type of commitment establishes an evidence-based culture of inquiry, innovation, and systems improvement [6]. Building APN capacity to conduct research sets the stage for the ongoing and evidence-based evolution of the APN role and for strengthening the position of APN roles as leaders for informing and driving healthcare innovation. (P. Harman, D. Bryant-Lukosius & R. Martin-Misener, CCAPNR, McMaster University, Canada, 30 March 2016, personal communication).

Conclusion

Provision of healthcare services by advanced practice nurses is reported as being valuable and effective but at times invisible as the impact on care specifically delivered by APNs is not highlighted nearly enough in research and publications. Focusing on APN-sensitive outcome indicators is vital for pointing out the presence and contributions of APNs. Continued attention to research that evaluates and describes APN roles plus evidence supporting best clinical practice is required. This expectation aligns with the call for APNs to acquire the knowledge base and skills to not only utilize research resources but also to participate in the research process and the implementation of research findings. This chapter describes the importance of APNs actively participating in the research process and identifies barriers that impede participation. A model that has successfully mentored research knowledge and skills for APNs concludes the chapter.

References

1. Bryant-Lukosius D (2015) Mentorship: a navigation strategy for promoting oncology nurse engagement in research. Can Oncol Nurs J 23(3):1–4
2. Bryant-Lukosius D, DiCenso A, Israr S, Charboneau-Smith R (2013) Resources to facilitate APN outcome research. In: Kleinpell R (ed) Outcome assessment in advanced practice nursing, 3rd edn. Springer Publishing Company, New York

3. Clarke S (2013) Practice-academia collaboration in nursing: contexts and future directions. Nurs Adm Q 37(3):184–193
4. De Palma JA (2009) Research. In: Hamric AB, Spross JA, Hanson CM (eds) Advanced nursing practice: an integrative approach, 4th edn. Saunders, St. Louis, pp 217–248
5. Fink R, Thompson C, Bonnes D (2005) Overcoming barriers and promoting the use of research in practice. J Nurs Adm 35(3):121–129
6. Harbman P, Bryant-Lukosius D, Martin-Misener R, Carter N, Covell C, Donald F, Gibbins S, Kilpatrick K, McKinlay J, Rawson K, Sherafali D, Tramner J, Valaitis R (under review) Partners in research: building academic-practice partnerships to educate and mentor advanced practice nurses
7. Houser J, Oman KS (2011) Evidence-based practice: an implementation guide for healthcare organizations. Jones & Bartlett, Sudbury
8. Kilpatrick K (2013) Understanding acute care nurse practitioner communication and decision-making in healthcare teams. J Clin Nurs 22(1–2):168–179
9. Kleinpell R, Alexandrov AW (2014) Integrative review of outcomes and performance improvement research on advanced practice nursing. In: Hamric AB, Hanson CM, Tracy MF, O'Grady ET (eds) Advanced practice nursing: an integrative approach. Elsevier Saunders, St. Louis, pp 607–644
10. Milner K (2015) Evidence-based practice. In: Stewart JG, Denisco SM (eds) Role development for the nurse practitioner. Jones & Bartlett, Burlington, pp 177–213
11. Pearson A, Wiechula R, Court A, Lockwood C (2005) The JBI model of evidence–based healthcare. Int J Evid Based Healthc 3(8):207–215. doi:10.1111/j.1479-6988.2005.00026.x
12. Tracy MF (2014) Direct clinical practice. In Hamric AB, Hanson CM, Tracy MF, O'Grady ET (eds) Advanced practice nursing: An integrative approach, 5th ed, pp. 147–182, Elsevier, St. Louis, MO

The Future: Strengthening the Advanced Nursing Practice Agenda

10

Abstract

Advanced Nursing Practice has become a well-established discipline internationally with an increasing presence noted in both developed and developing countries. This increased visibility places the evolving nature of ANP at a turning point. As an emerging and vital field of nursing in the healthcare workforce a look to the future implies a need to strengthen the focus on understanding the role and practice level of the advanced practice nurse. In addition, it is up to the profession to meet diverse worldwide healthcare challenges by developing pathways and services corresponding to countries' healthcare needs and resources. This chapter discusses aspects of preparing for a future healthcare workforce that increasingly includes advanced practice nurses providing care and healthcare services. Proposed topics to strengthen the international advanced nursing practice agenda are identified. Topics for the future include consensus building on terminology relevant to advanced nursing practice, workforce planning when integrating the levels of advanced nursing practice, capacity building by removing barriers to practice and enhancing the research agenda.

Keywords

Consensus • Terminology • Capacity building • Healthcare workforce • Removing barriers

Advanced Nursing Practice (ANP) has become a well-established discipline internationally with an increasing presence noted in both developed and developing countries. This increased visibility places the evolving nature of ANP at a turning point. As an emerging and vital field of nursing in the healthcare workforce a look to the future implies a need to strengthen the focus on understanding the role or level of the advanced practice nurse (APN). In addition, it is up to the profession to meet diverse worldwide healthcare challenges by developing pathways and services corresponding to countries' healthcare needs and resources. This chapter discusses aspects of preparing for a future healthcare workforce that increasingly includes

© Springer International Publishing Switzerland 2016
M. Schober, *Introduction to Advanced Nursing Practice*,
DOI 10.1007/978-3-319-32204-9_10

APNs providing care and healthcare services. Proposed topics to strengthen the international ANP agenda are identified. Topics for the future include consensus building on terminology relevant to ANP, workforce planning when integrating the levels of APN practice, capacity building by removing barriers to the full potential of advanced nursing practice and enhancing the research agenda.

10.1   National and International Organizational Views for the Future

The Institute of Medicine in the United States collaborated with the Robert Wood Johnson Foundation to conduct an investigation of the healthcare concerns of the country and the situation of nursing within the healthcare workforce. The resultant report [6] calls on nursing, individually and as a profession, to transform itself into a relevant force for solutions to meet the future healthcare needs of diverse populations. The report emphasized that nurses must be allowed to practice in ways that are consistent with their professional education and that the education they receive must better prepare them to deliver patient-centered, equitable, safe, high quality healthcare services. In referring specifically to APNs, a top recommendation is to remove scope of practice barriers to allow APNs to practice to the full extent of their education. In addition, the report concluded that the power for healthcare reform and change rests not only with nurses but also with governments, healthcare institutions, professional organizations, researchers, citizen advocacy groups, and other healthcare professionals.

The World Health Organization (WHO) emphasizes that nursing and midwifery delivery of services take place in partnership with other professionals and that future strategies should incorporate interprofessional education and collaborative practice. WHO also notes that removing barriers to practice and education can help nurses and midwives practice to the full extent of their education and training in order to address contemporary health challenges. Governments and relevant stakeholders should ensure that the nursing and midwifery workforce is appropriately prepared and enabled to practice to their full scope. It is on this platform that the WHO Strategic Directions for Nursing and Midwifery (SDNM) 2016–2020 is built [13]. Based on work done for previous SDNMs 2002–2008 and 2011–2015, these recommendations provide policymakers, practitioners, and other stakeholders at every level of the healthcare system with strategic directions for broad-based, collaborative action to enhance the capacity of nurses and midwives.

The strategic intent of the International Council of Nurses (ICN) 2014–2018 is to enhance the health of individuals, populations, and societies by (1) championing the contribution and image of nurses worldwide, (2) advocating for nurses at all levels, (3) advancing the nursing profession, and (4) influencing health, social, economic, and education policy [5]. As a federation of more than 130 national nursing associations, ICN represents more than 16 million nurses worldwide. The ever-increasing networks and global links provided by ICN reinforce the importance of connections with national, regional, and international nursing and nonnursing organizations. Building positive relationships internationally helps shape an agenda for the future of nursing including advanced nursing practice. As has been mentioned in earlier chapters, ICN has been instrumental in actively supporting and promoting an increased visibility for APN roles (see Chap. 2 for further discussion on international support for ANP and the ICN APN Network).

The attention by national and international organizations highlighting nursings' capacity to contribute to worldwide healthcare is noteworthy. However, this wide-ranging awareness mandates translation into a strategic agenda along with a call for APNs to step forward in a more influential and proactive manner. To facilitate this dialogue and promote action, the following sections provide topics to consider for the future.

10.2 Consensus Building Around Terminology

Literature and previous chapters in this monograph have underscored the substantial uncertainty, confusion, and ambiguity surrounding many features of ANP. The vagueness and lack of clarity has an effect on identification of titles, role definition, scopes of practice, standards for education, and policies meant to address APN practice. In addition, this uncertainty leads to a level of misunderstanding as to the APN role and its potential in the healthcare workforce. Lack of comprehension exists not only in geographical regions and from country to country but within countries as individuals and diverse entities attempt to interpret what advanced nursing or the advancement of nursing means in the provision of healthcare services. The dissimilarities are incompatible with a perspective that a systematic approach to ANP development internationally would be helpful, especially to those country initiatives that are in their infancy.

In an effort to provide a benchmark for international dialogue ICN has provided an APN definition, scope of practice, and characteristics [3,4]. Emphasizing that role development is sensitive to country context, this point of reference can be utilized by governments, institutions, countries, and regions in the process of realizing the complexities of ANP. The ICN definition and profile of ANP can be found in Chap. 1 (see also Sect. 1.1.3 for assumptions that form the foundation for ANP wherever nursing exists). In addition, Chap. 3 provides a discussion of titles, role characteristics, scope of practice, and competencies. Illustrations in Chap. 2 offer examples of how specific countries approached issues associated with terminology and definitions. A continued approach to some level of consensus building is imperative for the future.

As evidenced in the literature and this publication, the concept of consensus building is fraught with difficulties. The challenge is to identify effective and sustainable mechanisms that encourage periodic updating of an international focus around core components of the APN role and advanced level of practice. As a move to consensus building evolves, there is a need to acknowledge the diversity in nursing practice worldwide that has contributed and continues to contribute to a global identity for advanced nursing practice.

10.3   Integrating Advanced Nursing Practice into Healthcare Systems

As healthcare planners, policymakers, and administrators face the escalating challenges of providing cost-effective, accessible healthcare services, they are pursuing options for not only expanding hospital-based care but also strategies for becoming less reliant on the hospital sector. As mentioned earlier in this chapter, nurses and in particular nurses in advanced levels of practice and roles are in an ideal position to participate in reshaping healthcare strategies. This participation will likely include APNs as first point of contact in primary care, coordinating and managing care for chronic conditions and home care as well as establishing themselves as nurse entrepreneurs leading to a greater degree of independence in practice.

As evidenced in country scenarios and profiles in Chap. 2, healthcare reform and/or improved utilization of the nursing workforce has caught the attention of ministries of health and healthcare planners. Ideally, to approach workforce planning and inclusion of APN roles, a regulatory/legislative framework that includes title protection, scope of practice, and agreed to standards for education and practice needs to be in place. Planning and assessment of financial and human resources that coincide with establishing a framework can ensure that the APN will become not only successful but also a sustainable healthcare provider for the future. Examples of frameworks to review can be found in Chap. 5. See Chap. 6 for an in-depth discussion of professional regulation relevant to ANP.

National healthcare policies and priorities, the maturity of the nursing profession, access and basic preparation for advanced education, social trends, as well as funding sources will determine the rate or possibility of progression toward ANP. Research that provides evidence of the effectiveness of APNs in meeting health systems goals and champions that advocate for the creation of clinical positions as part of career pathways can strengthen the appeal for inclusion of APN roles [10].

10.4   Capacity Building

The increase in literature and publications associated with ANP implies an enthusiasm for capacity building activities related to nursing worldwide. Challenges and limitations have been discussed in earlier chapters. At times there is a lag between interest in implementing APN roles and establishing the foundation and processes that support such a change in the capacity of nurses to gain additional education plus function at a new level of nursing practice. However, to be clearly understood, capacity building refers not only to the individual but also to strengthening links and development in healthcare environments and within institutions to establish an environment conducive to advanced nursing practice. Capacity building optimally increases the range of people, organizations, and decision makers with the ability to identify concerns or problematic issues and develop solutions and subsequent actions.

For a strategic approach and a futuristic agenda, APNs and representatives of the ANP agenda must gain an understanding of the key roles of leaders within and outside of nursing as well as the nuances and complexities of making policy changes to remove regulatory and organizational obstructions in order to integrate APNs into the healthcare workforce. Capacity building for the future APN must include increasing the capacity to not only understand policy and the policy process but also attain the capability to produce appropriate, effective, sustainable strategies for implementing the policies for future healthcare professionals and systems.

An example of global nursing capacity building is provided by ICAP (access http://icap.columbia.edu/) with the implementation of the Global Nurse Capacity Building Program (GNCBP). Its aims are to improve population health by fostering individuals, institutions, and networks to expand, enhance, and sustain the nursing and midwifery workforce by achieving three objectives:

- Improve the quantity, quality, and relevance of nurses and midwives to address essential population-based healthcare needs, including HIV and other life-threatening conditions
- Identify, evaluate, and disseminate innovative human resource for health models and practices that are generalizable for national scale-up of nursing and midwifery education
- Build local and regional partnerships to provide technical and capacity building support for nursing and midwifery policy, regulatory and faculty development, curricula reform, continuing professional development and retention, and high impact nursing leadership

There appears to be a shortage of experienced, knowledgeable nurses capable of thinking and acting strategically and effectively in the policy and regulatory environment. The future for ANP requires increased capacity of nursing leaders to create sound models for APN practice and to set up APN services consistent with healthcare needs. This agenda item for the future invites the nursing profession to be both innovative and practical in participating in actions that increase the capacity of healthcare systems and the profession to promote ANP.

10.5 Additional Research

Although a core focus of ANP is clinical expertise, there is increasing emphasis on the development of a research component as a characteristic of ANP [1,7,9]. In addition, as mentioned earlier, as healthcare and reform in services evolves, the need to demonstrate the position and value of ANP is becoming increasingly important. In order to respond to the interest in clinical outcomes associated with APN services and confirm the diversity in APN roles, nurses practicing in advanced roles and advanced levels must develop a receptive attitude to the research process, participate in research, and document the research findings. Readily available evidence supporting the role is increasingly impor-tant as key stakeholders, decision makers, managers, administrators, and other healthcare professionals request data clarifying the role and clinical outcomes [8]. (see Chap. 9 for further discussion of research and Sect. 9.2.1 for a descrip-tion of The Canadian Centre for Advanced Practice Nursing Research (CCAPNR)).

As a unique and new professional in the healthcare workforce, the APN is increasingly called upon to portray a clear image of professional nursing as it is exhibited at an advanced level of practice. Not only is evidence and data helpful, but there is also a need to focus on aspects specific to APN practice rather than continually comparing APN practice to medical care. Outcomes and contributions of ANP need to be specifically attributed to the APN role to enhance the accuracy of research that is conducted [8]. All too often the impact of APNs is invisible in medically driven healthcare systems that lack ANP-sensitive indicators [1]. In the future, confirming the value ANP brings to healthcare will require specific and accurate appraisal of the healthcare delivery systems, settings, and structure in which they practice.

However, evidence in itself is not enough. As APNs increasingly participate in research, they will also be called upon to assess the quality of the research conducted and translate findings into practice. Even though overall research reporting on the impact of ANP is favorable, Kleinpell and Alexandrov [8] point out the need to be cautious in reviewing results as studies have the potential for respondent bias, questionable substantiation of what is reported and participants included in studies that are unfamiliar with the role and services being studied. In addition, if the APN of the future is expected to include research as a role component in clinical practice, they will be expected to optimally use and implement the evidence. Healthcare systems and employers will need to acknowledge that this is a legitimate component of the APN role and make provision accordingly, e.g., resources, access to research funding, recognition that research is part of the role, and time to conduct research projects (see Chap. 9 – Sect. 9.2.1 for a model of research mentorship). Gerrish et al [2] dem-onstrated that APNs are not only able to take up research but that they can be instrumental in "knowledge brokering" as a means of utilizing evidence in clini-cal settings with other nurses.

Even though international literature increasingly substantiates positive data sup-portive of ANP, the descriptions and evidence continue to mainly originate from developed countries and from those countries that have a longer history of success with APN roles. Chapter 2, in describing a growing presence of ANP, provides a glimpse of initiatives in their infancy from China, Kenya, Latin America, Oman, Pakistan, and South Africa; however, research describing the presence of ANP out-side of developed countries is scarce. Future research that includes a broad spectrum of countries has the potential of not only documenting outcomes but also comparing differences and similarities as to the motivation, development, and critical strategies relevant to advanced nursing roles. Research based on diverse development may confirm or reject the notion of possible consensus building around ANP as mentioned earlier in Sect. 10.2.

Conclusion

The prospects for advanced nursing practice to flourish in the future in diverse capacities worldwide are encouraging. This chapter discusses topics that require attention as this trend in professional nursing evolves. With increased attention from national and international organizations, ANP representatives and leaders will be called upon to a greater extent to provide a clearer profile of the ANP concept and its value to healthcare systems. From hospital-based positions to first point of service in primary care, evidence of practice outcomes and worth in healthcare provision continues to be needed to build a strong case supportive of the distinctive nature of ANP. Gaps in accessible education and opportunity for career progression exist thus reinforcing the urgent nature for capacity building. Finally, policies that limit and block APNs from practicing to their full potential require amendment and alteration. The agenda for the future is not only a challenge to forward thinking for nursing leaders but to others who acknowledge and support this dynamic change for the nursing profession.

References

1. Flanagan JM, Jones DA, Harris A (2013) Advanced practice registered nurses: accomplishments, trends, and future developments. In: Joel LA (ed) Advanced practice nursing: essentials for role development, 3rd edn. FA Davis, Philadelphia, pp 429–438
2. Gerrish K, McDonnell A, Nolan M, Guillaume L, Kirshbaum M, Tod A (2011) Factors influencing advanced practice nurses' ability to promote evidence-based practice among frontline nurses. Worldviews Evid Based Nurs 67(9):2004–2014. doi:10.1111/j.1365-2648.2011.05642.x
3. International Council of Nurses (ICN) (2002) Definition and characteristics of the role. http://www.icn-apnetwork.org. Accessed 19 Feb 2016
4. International Council of Nurses (ICN) (2008) The scope of practice, standards and competencies of the advanced practice nurse, ICN regulation series. International Council of Nurses, Geneva
5. International Council of Nurse (ICN) (2014–2018) http://www.icn.ch/images/stories/documents/about/ICN_Strategic_Plan.pdf. Accessed 15 May 2016
6. Institute of Medicine (IOM) (2011) The future of nursing: leading change, advancing health. The National Academies Press, Washington, DC
7. Kilpatrick K, Harbman P, Carter N, Martin-Misener R, Bryant-Lukosius D, Donald F, Kaasalainen S, Bourgeault I, DiCenso A (2010) The acute care nurse practitioner role in Canada. Can J Nurs Leadersh 23(Special Issue):115–139
8. Kleinpell R, Alexandrov AW (2014) Integrative review of outcomes and performance improvement research on advanced practice nursing. In: Hamric AB, Hanson CM, Tracy MF, O'Grady ET (eds) Advanced practice nursing: an integrative approach, 5th edn. Elsevier Saunders, St. Louis, pp 607–644
9. McGee P (2009) The future of advanced practice. In: McGee P (ed) Advanced practice in nursing and the allied health professions, 3rd edn. Wiley-Blackwell, Oxford, pp 243–254

10. Schober M (2013) Factors influencing the development of advanced practice nursing in Singapore. Doctoral thesis, Sheffield Hallam University, Sheffield Hallam University archives. http://shura.shu.ac.uk/7799/17. Accessed May 2016
11. Villeneuve M, MacDonald J (2006) Toward 2020: visions for nursing. Canadian Nurses Association, Ottawa
12. World Health Organization (WHO) (2010) Strategic directions for strengthening nursing and midwifery services 2011–2015. WHO, Geneva. Access from http://www.who.int/hrh/nursing_midwifery/en/
13. World Health Organization (WHO) (2015) Strategic directions for strengthening nursing and midwifery services 2016–2020. WHO, Geneva. Access from http://www.who.int/hrh/nursing_midwifery/en/

Index

© Springer International Publishing Switzerland 2016
M. Schober, *Introduction to Advanced Nursing Practice*,
DOI 10.1007/978-3-319-32204-9